Antiracist
Occupational Therapy

of related interest

Supporting Trans People of Colour
How to Make Your Practice Inclusive
Sabah Choudrey
ISBN 978 1 78775 059 3
eISBN 978 1 78775 060 9

White Privilege Unmasked
How to be Part of the Solution
Judy Ryde
ISBN 978 1 78592 408 8
eISBN 978 1 78450 767 1

Overcoming Everyday Racism
Building Resilience and Wellbeing in the Face
of Discrimination and Microaggressions
Susan Cousins
ISBN 978 1 78592 850 5
eISBN 978 1 78592 851 2

Being White in the Helping Professions
Developing Effective Intercultural Awareness
Judy Ryde
ISBN 978 1 84310 936 5
eISBN 978 1 84642 730 5

Antiracist Occupational Therapy

Unsettling the Status Quo

Edited by
Musharrat J. Ahmed-Landeryou
Foreword by Professor Elelwani Ramugondo

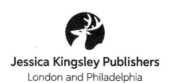

Jessica Kingsley Publishers
London and Philadelphia

First published in Great Britain in 2024 by Jessica Kingsley Publishers
An imprint of John Murray Press

I

A CIP catalogue record for this title is available from the
British Library and the Library of Congress

ISBN 978 1 83997 574 5
eISBN 978 1 83997 575 2

Printed and bound in Great Britain by CPI Group

Jessica Kingsley Publishers' policy is to use papers that are natural,
renewable and recyclable products and made from wood grown in
sustainable forests. The logging and manufacturing processes are expected
to conform to the environmental regulations of the country of origin.

Jessica Kingsley Publishers
Carmelite House
50 Victoria Embankment
London EC4Y 0DZ

www.jkp.com

John Murray Press
Part of Hodder & Stoughton Ltd
An Hachette Company

In memory of George Perry Floyd Jnr.
(1973–2020)

Contents

Contributors

Kosiwa Lokosu, Sihle Mwela, Professor Roshan Galvaan, Lily Owens, Shahedah Vawda, Kalimah Ibrahiim, Kwaku Agyemang, Fasloen Adams, Dr Khalilah Robinson Johnson PhD, Dr Selena Washington PhD, Eric Nkansah Opoku, Dr Ellen Serwaa Adomako PhD, Sherrille Tayson, Oliver Miller, Valentine Tendai Mutsvairo, Musharrat J. Ahmed-Landeryou, Peter Bredu-Darkwa, Isla Emery-Whittington, Jaime Daniel Leite Junior, Sheela Ivlev, Dr Ryan Lavalley PhD, Dr Marie-Lyne Grenier PhD, Kirsty Stanley, David Marsden, Dr Magno Nunes Farias PhD, Odeth Richardson

Foreword

Health professionals who are deeply aware of systems of oppression understand wounds that find expression through ill-health; wounds that emanate from intergenerational trauma, often triggered and sustained by systemic and structural racism. Key to this is that racial oppression always intersects with other forms of oppression around language, nationality, ethnicity, gender, religion, class, functional variability, as well as sexual identity. When health professionals are Black and brown individuals, and recognize these wounds in themselves and others, but find courage to give voice to these lived experiences, perhaps only then can the world begin to heal. Courage in this speaks to the fact that these individuals have always had to fight against historically sustained resistance to get their voices heard.

It comes as no surprise, therefore, that this book is one of its kind in occupational therapy to date. To edit and author a book through a mainstream publisher, in the predominantly white occupational therapy literature, as a collective of mostly Black and brown people from around the world, and naming racism as the elephant in the room, is unprecedented in the history of the profession.

Black and brown people are often spoken for, about and over; they are reduced to objects of analysis on oppression, never seen as subjects who can analyse their own situations. This book disrupts this practice in the profession and is a welcome example of how to theorise present struggle from a place of racial oppression, speaking from within a discipline in health. Now that these Black and brown professionals in occupational therapy, globally, have spoken – have dared to speak out – the classic question will arise from potential allies who do not share the body-biographical-geo-political epistemic positionalities of most of the authors: what about me and what can I do? The answer to this is a set of questions: are you willing to co-exist with Black and brown people as fully deserving human beings? What in Black and brown people co-existing on their own terms unsettles you the most and why? How have you engaged with your own history and colonial tendencies that continue? What is your role in co-creating dependency, predicated on the superiority-inferiority racial dynamic?

Professor Elelwani Ramugondo, DVC Transformation, Student Affairs & Social Responsiveness, University of Cape Town, South Africa

Acknowledgements

High gratitude to:

My daughter and husband, without whose support and unmeasurable understanding, I cannot continue this all-consuming and thankless but necessary work of antiracism activism in occupational therapy. Everyone doing this work needs the unconditional love and compassion of their family to keep going – it was the same for me.

The contributors of the book for their motivation and passion for antiracism to be embedded in occupational therapy – without them we would not have a book.

BAMEOTUK and DISRUPTOT who are my light in the dark and hope of future change for antiracism, equity and justice in occupational therapy. Special shout out to Ed Sum from BAMEOTUK, who helped through some very low times in the struggle for antiracism.

LGBTQIA+OTUK and AbleOTUK, two affinity groups formed after BAMEOTUK which have improved my feelings of belonging in occupational therapy. Some members have explicitly shown solidarity in times when I have struggled.

Preface

In 2020, with the increasing pain, disappointment and frustration I was feeling with the occupational therapy profession, I needed outlets that would lead to collaboration with other people. This book is one of the many outlets I found. It continues the social movement for change and accountability for occupational therapy to not just be antiracist[1] but to action antiracism in an impactful and sustainable manner. This book is challenging the widely accepted Eurocentric notions embedded in occupational therapy and occupational science, by starting to interrogate them. This book is only a starting point.

Imperialism is the conceptualisation of policies regarding political suppression, economic suppression and knowledge suppression typically carried out by a country from the Global North on another country usually from the Global South, and colonialism is the enaction of the policies. The colonising country justifies its actions and keeps control through socially constructed policies on racial hierarchy, wealth, land and other distribution of resources, and indigenous knowledge suppression and ways of being (Quijano 2000). This in turn is carried on today, as coloniality, where mainly Black and minoritised persons are continually held up against the colonial yardstick of what is considered normal: white, male, English speaking, Christian, heterosexual, able-bodied, upper/middle class, and so on. The data shows that the outcome of health inequities is the result of white supremacy in health and social care organisations, and occupational therapy is part of these organisations. Remember, you don't have to be racialised as white to reproduce

---

[1] Antiracist/antiracism is used by the authors; it is a political stance of protest and opposition, to be actively acting against racism, in that being anti to racism is not an add on or opposite to racism. 'In a *racist* society, it is *not* enough to be *non-racist*, we must be *antiracist*' (Prof. Angela Y. Davis, cited in Rutherford 2020: 185).

and uphold white supremacy, as the colonialist mindset is the default in society and thus gets translated into action. Occupational therapy is a profession conceived by white people for white people. The Eurocentric bias of occupational therapy philosophy, knowledge and education has been reproduced globally. Frustratingly, even in the literature referenced for chapters of this book, the authorship is primarily white.

It is not good enough to only roll out Black and brown individuals for leadership when it comes to antiracism or equality, diversity and inclusion initiatives and changes. It is not for the Black and brown bodies in the profession, the communities we collaborate with and the service users who come to us to be doing the heavy lifting of antiracism change-making in the profession. They did not construct racism and they do not benefit from racial capital. Why aren't individuals from racialised, minoritised, under-represented and marginalised groups more visible and frequently represented in the diversity of leadership roles/positions? We know that a diverse team enhances employees' innovation and creations, and service user and employee satisfaction, and hence improves and benefits organisations.

Occupational therapy professional bodies, professionals, educators and students need to stop hiding behind inaction, sound bites and metaphors, and actively follow through on the social justice foundations the profession claims to be built on. Occupational therapy needs to urgently integrate and embed antiracism in its principles, processes and practices, actively and explicitly.

All the contributors are cognizant that they are in a privileged position to be able to write for this book and then to have a publisher agree to take on the content and disseminate it. We treat the power that comes from the privilege to be able to write this book with respect, and call on the occupational therapy communities to collaborate in this work. I can't bring about antiracism change in the profession on my own; Black and brown bodies can't do it on their own. To disrupt the continuing institutional racism and microaggression in our profession, we need to be large, coordinated action global collaboratives that cannot be ignored.

Let's unsettle occupational therapy and make it contemporary, globally representative and antiracist. Let's get on with actions now, not later.

Purpose of the book

The book is a collaboration of some BAMEOTUK network members, and national and international peers and allies. The content does not dilute or hide the context of the countries that the contributors are writing from. I envisioned this book as a gathering to amplify rather than diminish the voices that want to challenge the status quo of Eurocentric dominance of occupational therapy. As a book that could be read by anyone, whether they be the public, our service users, or allied health or anyone in health and social care, this book could be on their bookshelves to refer to when developing antiracist approaches for education, policies and service delivery. This book brings together topics to elucidate racism in occupational therapy from different perspectives and support actions for antiracism in the profession. It is innovative, open and unique in bringing together the topics it addresses for occupational therapy, but also in that it is based not just on literature evidence but on lived experiences too. At the end of each chapter there is a quadrant reflection log to help you to pause, reflect on and summarise your learning, and to identify actions to realistically employ what you take from each chapter. A template for the quadrant reflection log is available to download at www.jkp.com/catalogue/book/9781839975745.

Hold yourself to account to enact antiracist occupational therapy every day.

Musharrat J. Ahmed-Landeryou, editor

Chapter Summary and Contributors

Chapter 1: Introduction – Setting the Scene of Unrest
This chapter introduces the factors that led to the 2020 global resurgence of focus on racism and health inequalities/inequities and why it matters to the occupational therapy community.

Kosiwa Lokosu, BSc (Hons) Occupational Therapy, specialist occupational therapist, UK

Sihle Mwela, BSc (Hons) Occupational Therapy, specialist occupational therapist for East London NHS Foundation Trust, UK

Professor Roshan Galvaan, Faculty of Health Sciences Division of Occupational Therapy, University of Cape Town, South Africa

Chapter 2: Introduction to Critical Race Theory
This chapter introduces the reader to the concept of critical race theory and its relevance to occupational therapy.

Lily Owens, BSc (Hons) Occupational Therapy, PgCert, MA Ed, senior occupational therapist and educator, Wales; independent researcher, Swansea University, Wales, UK

Shahedah Vawda, BA (Hons) Occupational Therapy, PGCHE occupational therapist (clinician and teacher), Bridges Associate Trainer, UK

Chapter 3: Contribution of Racism in Racial Inequalities, Health Inequities and Social Determinants of Health and Occupational Therapy

This chapter critically discusses how and why racism is contributing to inequities on a population level in healthcare, and relates this to occupational therapy.

Kalimah Ibrahiim, BA (Hons), BSc (Hons), MPH, MRCOT, FRSPH, Senior Lecturer, Admissions Lead and Course Leader for the BSc Occupational Therapy course, University of East London, UK

Kwaku Agyemang, Occupational Therapist Prison Services, and co-founder of BAMEOTUK, UK

Dr Fasloen Adams, BA Occupational Therapy, MSc Occupational Therapy, PhD BOT (SU), MScOT (UCT), PhD (Wits), Senior Lecturer, Division of Occupational Therapy Department, Department of Health and Rehabilitation Sciences, Faculty of Medicine and Health Sciences, Stellenbosch University, South Africa

Chapter 4: Antiracist Occupational Therapy Education: Perspectives from Ghana, the United Kingdom and the United States of America

This chapter discusses why antiracist approaches to curricula could contribute to action in disrupting western centric dominance of occupational therapy education and hence practice.

Dr Khalilah Robinson Johnson, PhD, MS, OTR/L, Assistant Professor, Division of Occupational Science and Occupational Therapy, University of North Carolina at Chapel Hill, United States

Dr Selena Washington, PhD, MSPH, OTR/L, Assistant Professor, Saint Louis University, United States

Eric Nkansah Opoku, BSc (Hons) Occupational Therapy, MSc Occupational Therapy, Senior Research Assistant/Clinical Placement Coordinator, Department of Occupational Therapy, University of Ghana [at time of writing]

Dr Ellen Serwaa Adomako, Lecturer, University of Essex, UK

Chapter 5: Experiences of Racism in Occupational Therapy Clinical Placement Settings

The chapter provides insight of racism for Black students on placement through stories of experiences, and potential actions for education for practice educators.

Sherrille Tayson, occupational therapist, UK [student at time of writing]

Oliver Miller, BSc, community occupational therapist, UK

Valentine Tendai Mutsvairo, MSc Occupational Therapy, BSc (Hons), occupational therapist, sport and exercise science, UK

Musharrat J. Ahmed-Landeryou, SFHEA, MSc Clinical Neurosciences, CLTHE, Licentiate TCM Acupuncture, (BSc Hons) Occupational Therapy, BSc (Hons) Physics with Med. Applic., Associate Professor, London South Bank University. Co-founder of BAMEOTUK, PhD research student at time of writing, UK

Chapter 6: Ethnic Neutral Occupational Therapy Services in Health and Social Care Contribute to Maintaining Structural Inequity

This chapter critically explores the history and current consequences of ethnic neutrality in occupational therapy practice and services and offers a guidance on how to sustainably change.

Musharrat J. Ahmed-Landeryou, SFHEA, MSc Clinical Neurosciences, CLTHE, Licentiate TCM Acupuncture, (BSc Hons) Occupational Therapy, BSc (Hons) Physics with Med. Applic., Associate Professor, London South Bank University. PhD student at time of writing, UK

Peter Bredu-Darkwa, BSc (Hons) Occupational Therapy, Mphil, Disability, Rehabilitation and Development. Lecturer/Health Tutor, Accra School of Hygiene/University of Ghana

Chapter 7: Antiracism as Means and Ends

This chapter argues why and how measures of antiracism require nothing less than the collaborative strength of collectives and outlines a stepwise antiracism programme as a way forward.

Isla Emery-Whittington, PhD candidate, Kaupapa Māori researcher, occupational therapist, SHORE Whariki Research Centre, Massey University, Auckland, Aotearoa, New Zealand

Jaime Daniel Leite Junior, occupational therapist, PhD student. Member of the Metuia Network, Social Occupational Therapy; SexGen-OTOS: International Network on Sexualities and Genders within Occupational Therapy and Occupational Science; Dona Ivone Lara Group: Occupational Therapy and Black Population, Brazil

Sheela Ivlev, occupational therapist, DisruptOT founder, United States

Chapter 8: Active Antiracist Allyship in Occupational Therapy

This chapter offers an exploration as to what it means to be in active solidarity in becoming an ally who racialized as white – the pitfall, challenges and ways to be an active ally.

Dr Ryan Lavalley, PhD, OTR/L, Assistant Professor, University of North Carolina at Chapel Hill, United States

Dr Marie-Lyne Grenier, MScOT, DOT, PhD(c), erg., Canada

Kirsty Stanley, BSc (Hons) Occupational Therapy, Director, Occupational Therapist and Writer at Occupation4Life Ltd, UK

David Marsden, BSc (Hons) Occupational Therapy, MSc, UK

Chapter 9: Going Forwards

This chapter discusses how we know what we know and how we move forward and act.

Dr Magno Nunes Farias, OT, MSc, PhD, Adjunct Professor at the University of Brasília, Faculty of Ceilândia (UnB-FCE/Brazil). Member of the Metuia Network, Social Occupational Therapy; SexGen-OTOS: International Network on Sexualities and Genders within Occupational Therapy and Occupational Science; Dona Ivone Lara Group: Occupational Therapy and Black Population, Brazil

Odeth Richardson, BSc Occupational Therapy, MSc Clinical Leadership, Head of Service Occupational Therapy at The Newcastle Upon Tyne Hospitals NHS Foundation Trust, Chair of Royal College of Occupational Therapists, UK

References

References from all the chapters are collated for your convenience at the end of the book.

CHAPTER 1

Introduction – Setting the Scene of Unrest

Kosiwa Lokosu, Sihle Mwela, Professor Roshan Galvaan

For a profession built on principles of person-centredness, empowerment, justice and human rights (World Federation of Occupational Therapists (WFOT) 2019; Royal College of Occupational Therapists (RCOT) 2021a; WFOT 2021), there appears to have been little representation of racism and health inequalities/inequities within the occupational therapy literature (Bass-Haugen 2009). Racism and health inequalities/inequities systemically impact the very populations we work with and belong to (Marmot *et al.* 2020a, 2020b; WFOT 2020), hence, it is important to examine the fundamentals of occupational therapy against these and consider what this holds for current and future practice. We are living at a time where accountability is being raised more frequently because social and institutional responsibility repeatedly fails, especially when political, institutional and social issues are everybody's business and duty. If in doubt whether racism is a topic for occupational therapy, read the outcomes of Beagan *et al.*'s (2022) qualitative research on systemic racism in Canadian occupational therapy or the scoping review from Sterman and Njelesani (2021) 'Becoming anti-racist occupational therapy practitioners'; and another a continuing professional development paper for the American Occupational Therapy Association by Lucas and Washington (2020) on 'Understanding Systemic Racism in the United States: Educating Our Students and Ourselves'. These papers, and others, are telling the profession that racism exists in the profession and we need to deal with it to be able to genuinely and credibly offer equitable services to all those we work with and alongside. Racism is power imbalance (Kendi 2019), and by not addressing racism in occupational therapy we maintain this power imbalance and continue to support and contribute to the status quo of institutional racism in health and social care. We cannot wait any longer for the profession and professionals of occupational therapy to be actively antiracist; this resonates with James Baldwin's call to action when he states:

> What is it you wanted me to reconcile myself to? I was born here almost 60 years ago. I'm not going to live another 60 years. You've always told me 'it takes time'. It's taken my father's time, my mother's time, my uncles' time, my brothers' and my sisters' time, my nieces' and nephews' time. How much time do you want for your progress? (American Masters 1989)

This chapter introduces the factors that led to the 2020 global resurgence of focus on racism and health inequalities/inequities. As we explore these factors it may lead to questioning whether impactful strategies and actions have been implemented to disrupt the outcomes of decades of racism and classism.

The chapter is organised to answer the following critical questions:

- Why in 2020 was there a resurgence of focus on racism and health inequalities/inequities?

- What has been done so far to tackle racism and health inequalities in the occupational therapy profession?

COVID-19 pandemic

We have heard the suggestion that the COVID-19 pandemic was a societal leveller because it was indiscriminate in who succumbed to death from it. This indeed may be true, but it is not the truth. History repeatedly identifies that those who are most negatively impacted during pandemics and periods of societal unrest and struggle are the already minoritised and disadvantaged populations (Bambra *et al.* 2020). Public Health England (2020b: 6) identified that

> after accounting for the effect of sex, age, deprivation and region, people of Bangladeshi ethnicity had around twice the risk of death than people of white British ethnicity. People of Chinese, Indian, Pakistani, other Asian, Black Caribbean and other Black heritages, had between 10 and 50% higher risk of death when compared to white British.

This was further supported by more research which found that in mortality rates of healthcare professionals, a total of 63 per cent general staff, 64 per cent nursing staff and 94 per cent medical staff deaths in their groups were of Black, Asian and minoritised backgrounds (Cook *et al.* 2020). The UK mental health charity Mind (2020) completed a survey of over 14,000 adults and the results revealed that during the COVID-19 pandemic existing inequalities and inequities in healthcare, employment, finances and housing, among other concerns, had a greater impact on the mental health of individuals from different Black and minoritised communities compared to people who identify as racialised as white [will hereafter be referred to as white people] (Mind 2020). Furthermore, it is known that Black people in England are four times more likely to be detained under the Mental Health Act than white people (NHS Digital 2022). It is already documented that Black women are four times more likely to die in childbirth than their white counterparts; women who live in more deprived areas are three times more likely to die than those in the most affluent areas and as we know, people from Black and minoritised backgrounds are more likely to have poor socio-economic status (Limb 2021). Unfortunately, the same health inequalities/ inequities due to systemic racism and discrimination can be seen in other countries, such as Canada, with indigenous communities facing occupational injustice when trying to access medical services (Rammohan 2019). In Canada, there needs to be recognition of the violence, disappearances and the legacy of historical harm (Rammohan 2019). The continuation of systemic racism and discrimination shows little learning and advancement from past harms and significant historical events such as colonialism, settler colonialism and Apartheid.

For England, Marmot *et al.* (2020a) place the blame of these health inequalities and inequities as outcomes of systemic racism, and political inertia with chronic under-investment when it comes to health and social care by the Conservative government since it came into power in 2010. The pandemic undeniably spotlighted the pre-existing racism resulting in health inequalities and inequities experienced by Black and minoritised communities (Public Health England 2020a). Black and minoritised groups are essentially at a disadvantage every time they step out of the door due to the outcomes of systems pre-designed to disadvantage and exclude them and advance white supremacy. The new interest in racism, wider health determinants and wellbeing seems driven by concerns over the bruised economy, media and public pressure, which raises concern whether this is another temporary and transient moment in time with hope and potential for change (Oliver 2021). Such societal episodes appear to end in returning to the status quo, because maybe for people in power and advantage, antiracism change may feel as if their privilege will be lessened or is under attack and therefore they will be worse off.

George's public murder, 25 May 2020

On the evening of that tragic day, George Floyd, a 46-year-old father, son, brother, friend and family man, had gone to a local shop he frequented to buy cigarettes. The owner of the shop called him a friendly regular, but that evening the owner was not at the shop, and the person who was on the till called the police, suspecting a fake $20 from George. He wanted George to return the cigarettes but he refused. Derek Chauvin, the Minneapolis policeman, was found guilty of the manslaughter of George when he knelt on George's neck compressing it for 9 minutes and 29 seconds, even though George was restrained. George showed his distress by repeatedly saying 'I can't breathe' until he lost consciousness; Chauvin continued to kneel on George's neck for another minute after the ambulance came (Douglas *et al.* 2021).

It became a narrative of 'not another Black person being killed by the police' and brought further attention to the inequalities and inequities faced by the Black populations, initially in the United States then worldwide, regarding political disinterest in tackling systemic racism. While we have seen reoccurring protests every time a Black person is murdered by the police, this was different as not only were Black people suffering the impact of COVID-19 on their health and jobs, but they were also suffering at the hands of police, and systemic brutality in general set up against Black citizens – and the brutality was now filmed. The filmed video brought attention to the #BlackLivesMatter movement, which focuses on decentralising political control of United States police and transforming funding that is received by United States police to disrupt the police brutality and systemic anti-Black racism (Crowe 2018; Rojas 2020).

In response to the murder of George Floyd we repeatedly heard the phrases 'Black Lives Matter' and 'No Justice, No Peace' from the Black

Lives Matter (BLM) movement. The BLM movement was formed in 2013 following the death of Trayvon Martin in 2012 and the acquittal of his murderer George Zimmerman (Garza 2014). The BLM movement's United States founders are Alicia Garza, Patrisse Cullors and Opal Tometi (Garza 2014; Howard University 2018). The movement has grown in momentum following further tragic United States murders of Black lives such as Michael Brown, Sandra Bland, Eric Garner, Philando Castile, Alton Sterling, Breonna Taylor, along with many others. The intention of the BLM founders was that the movement would combat anti-Black policy and brutality and make visible the unacceptable maintained discrimination, disadvantage and racism Black people face daily (Garza 2014; Hordge-Freeman & Loblack 2020). BLM has become an official organisation, Black Lives Matter Global Network Foundation Inc., a social and decentralised political movement to eliminate systemic white supremacy and build local communities to intervene against violence and oppression on Black communities by the state and other groups (Blacklivesmatter.com 2020). Anti-Black racism, as the setting up of the global network suggests, is not just an issue within the United States, but is relevant in other countries, such as the UK, where we remember, for example, Mark Duggan, Joy Gardner, Habib Ullah, Christopher Alder, Sean Rigg and Chris Kaba – all UK citizens from Black and minoritised backgrounds whose deaths were at the hands of white UK police officers.

Over the years, this has become a matter of concern for more than just the Black, minoritized and indigenous communities. With the power of social media, the awareness of the BLM movement has become something that is widely talked about and recognised; it has moved out into the streets and into spaces Black people have not been allowed in before. The key concept to remember is that '#BlackLivesMatter doesn't mean your life isn't important – it means that Black lives, which are seen as without value within white supremacy, are important to your liberation' (Garza 2014). BLM is more than racism. It recognises the need for systemic change to social justice and the need for reform for transformation. It highlights the years of social, economic, physical and emotional disadvantages that marginalised and minoritised communities have faced and continue to face. The BLM organisation mentions that white supremacy reflects 'white centring' or white privilege'; the latter term was developed by sociologist W.E.B. Dubois in 1935 and describes the advantages and opportunities that are afforded automatically without effort due to having a white racial identity (Myers 2017). In her book, Reni Eddo-Lodge (2018) states that white privilege does not mean that people who racially identify as white do not experience discrimination, disadvantage or oppression, but rather that, if you are white or perceived as being white, this will positively affect your life (Eddo-Lodge 2018).

The year 2020 saw unprecedented times in which we all witnessed and lived through significant event after event. This included the coronavirus pandemic, the televised public witnessing of the murder of George Floyd, demonstrating blatant police brutality, the reprisal against this and political changes both in the UK and across the world promoting white supremacy. This feels like a pivotal time in history.

Having discussed the role of the COVID-19 pandemic and the BLM movement, we can see that it is not just one individual factor that contributed to the resurgence of focus around racism and health inequalities and inequities, but a multitude of various long-term, sustained factors interweaving with one another and making a barrier to antiracism change.

What has been done so far to tackle racism and health inequalities in the occupational therapy profession?

It has taken 104 years for the occupational therapy profession to take notice of the impact that racism has on those who practise the profession and those who receive its services (Kronenberg 2020b). We don't want to minimize the work that has led up to the racial reckoning that is long overdue but note that Black, minoritised and indigenous activists have never ceased to address racial injustices; it just took all this time for the occupational therapy community to notice and care. Our profession is purported to be built on the principles of the literature in occupational science and education on tackling racism and health inequalities, which should assist practitioners, educators and students in focusing on how to disrupt and address these (Simaan 2020a; Sterman & Njelesani 2021). A fundamental premise of occupational science and therapy is that participation in occupation can affect health and wellbeing; occupational justice is underpinned by a belief in the human right to engage in diverse and meaningful occupations to meet people's individual needs and develop their potential to thrive, not just survive (Wilcock & Townsend 2000). Thinking about social and occupational justice; social justice is essentially a view that there should be 'a balance between the people and its society where economic, social and political opportunities are available to all' (Braveman & Suarez-Balcazar 2009: 13). Although usually considered a part of social justice, occupational justice focuses on the 'right for everyone to have their basic needs met and be given equal opportunities and life chances to reach their potential engagement in diverse and meaningful occupation' (Wilcock & Townsend 2009: 193). As occupational therapists, we strive for people to have access to meaningful lives, but this is not always possible due to the structural limitations that impact minoritised populations, which result in othering, alienation, exclusion, maintenance of under-development and many more restrictions (Townsend & Wilcock 2004a). The quote by Braveman and Bass-Haugen, (2009: 11) best summarises the advice to the occupational therapy community:

> Social justice issues and health disparities are endemic and critical areas of national and global concern; their vastness is beyond the reach of any single discipline or profession, including occupational therapy. Engaging communities, professionals, researchers, educators, leaders, and policy makers from all disciplines is required to achieve our collective goals for a just society.

The factors that result in occupational injustice, health inequities and racism and actions for change in the profession are further explored in the chapters of this book.

As a profession, we should be concerned with police brutality, racism and health inequities as these affect our service users, their families and communities and their occupations. Health and social care is political (Borrell et al. 2007). The word politics comes from the Greek term *polis* which means city/state; *politeuma* is a body made from the community that deliberates on the good for the community and doing good for the community (local council/government), and *politeia* is translated as the way the community functions in everyday life in line with their moral beliefs; the citizens take part in looking after the city and each other (Miller 1980). Hence occupational therapy is political as it is in the business of health and social care and the health and wellbeing of the 'citizens' of the community, so as a profession it should be identifying, understanding and actively involved in all environmental change to enable individuals and communities to thrive – even if it also means being involved in local, regional and national politics for social justice, and therefore occupational justice. As a profession, we are not explicitly demonstrating and publicising our commitment and actions to disrupt racism, and disrupt the institutional racism of professional bodies and services for the benefit of service users and occupational therapy staff. We also fail in our responsibilities to disrupt structural barriers to occupational opportunities needed to target the systemic problems resulting in racism and health inequalities/inequities (Williams & Purdie-Vaughns 2016; Whalley Hammell 2017). This position is exacerbated by professional bodies being mostly silent or inactive when it comes to these issues. As occupational therapists, we are supposed to work with communities, populations and society to promote and enable equality of outcomes, equity in opportunities and access to services as human rights (Braveman & Bass-Haugen 2009).

In the UK, ironically all correspondence so far from the Royal College of Occupational Therapists (RCOT) has been enabled due to pressure applied by independent groups like BAMEOTUK Network, a campaigning pressure group of Black Asian and minoritised students, staff and educators collaborating to disrupt institutional racism in the profession. The BAMEOTUK Network called for the RCOT and occupational therapy professionals to be held accountable for their actions in their practice and everyday life regarding antiracism. People were recognising that the configuration of the RCOT and its membership was not reflective of Black Asian and minoritised populations, and RCOT members were vocalising their desire for change. Open letters were written to the RCOT from BAMEOTUK network members and allies, which asked for answers and challenged the status quo of keeping silent and carrying on the same approach from the RCOT, recycling the status quo of institutional racism (BAMEOTUK 2020; Occupational Therapy Magazine 2020). Dialogue between the RCOT and BAMEOTUK has resulted in an equality, diversity and inclusion (EDI) lead position to be created in the organisation and the position has been filled by Ketan Davé. The development of BAMEOTUK resulted in two other occupational therapy affinity groups to be formed in the UK due to ongoing inequities, LGBTQIA+OTUK and ABLEOTUK. Furthermore, since the formation of BAMEOTUK, the new elected chair of council, Odeth Richardson, is the first Black person to hold that position. However, there is still more to be done, with the RCOT collaborating with the affinity groups in disrupting institutional racism and discrimination in the profession and further, which has only just started.

As occupational therapy is a predominately white middle-class profession in general, it is the responsibilities of the occupational therapy professional bodies to educate themselves and guide and support students, practitioners and educators in learning about institutional racism in health and social care and the profession's behaviour in contributing to this, and in identifying impactful ways in which occupational therapy and science can disrupt this. Professor David Williams (2019) says that racism sets inflammatory responses in the body that lead to many different illnesses, meaning that racism is adding to the burden of healthcare. Moreover, the recent Lancet Review series (2022) articles add further credence to Professor Williams' research outcomes. It is our duty as occupational therapists to identify and address racism. There is a shared responsibility for all in the profession, not just for the Black, Asian and minoritised members, to ensure that we are providing the best and equitable care for our service users and peers (Lavalley & Robinson Johnson 2022).

It is unfortunate that many countries are in different phases, not only of awareness and willingness, but in having political influence to take action on the problems of racism and inequities in health that we see today (Mackenbach & Bakker 2003). The World Health Assembly of 1998 developed the Health 21 strategy, which aimed at improving health for all in the 21st century. Its second target, although ambitious, was that 'by the year 2020, the health gap between socio-economic groups within countries should be reduced by at least one quarter in all Member States, by substantially improving the health of disadvantaged groups' (World Health Organisation 1999: 16). Having reached the deadline, today we find that most countries are unable to bridge the gap, with the UK being among them. Historically, the UK has always had difficulty in acting on the given issues, with little push for policies that direct equitable access to care, treatment and health outcomes. As occupational therapists, our role is about empowering and enabling occupational participation, not only in the face of social determinants, race and health inequalities/ inequities, but in disrupting these factors through the profession's work. This is a difficult task without political willingness, money and resources, as it requires leaders and boards to change the culture of racism and inequalities through role-modelling antiracist behaviour and putting in place policies and measures to hold people to account (Kline 2020). We cannot wait for another generation to eradicate the problem of racism and health inequities, we need tangible and measurable policies sooner rather than later that change the impact for minoritised and marginalised people. Only that shift will end the persistent culture of racism and health inequalities and inequities (Moorley *et al.* 2020).

In South Africa, the occupational injustice is clear. As a result of the continuing fallout from Apartheid's past, the majority of individuals and communities who access public healthcare services are uninsured and living in deprived communities where access to basic necessities such as water, electricity and housing is scarce (Richards & Galvaan 2018). Research highlights the need for therapists to develop better understanding and awareness of the inequalities and inequities people face to allow recognition of how this affects their ability to meaningfully participate with occupation (Richards & Galvaan 2018). This enables the therapists to co-produce culturally relevant therapy and improve therapeutic relationships to enable self-identified success.

It is important, now more than ever, for organisations like occupational therapy professional bodies (such as the RCOT, the American Occupational Therapy Association or the Canadian Association of Occupational Therapists) to take note of what is happening today in our society and see how this affects the minoritised and marginalised populations – in violent and fatal consequences – and act impactfully to disrupt the status quo. It is important for professional bodies to now consider the institutional racism that occurs not just in the judicial system, police force, schooling system and more, but in their own organisations. How are their policy processes and practices impacting their own members? How do their Black and minoritised members continue to be under-represented and kept mainly in the margins, and feel a lack of belonging because of the racism they experience in the profession? Some occupational therapy professional bodies are on the edges of the path to change their culture and traditions. For example, the RCOT which, due to the pressure put on it from the BAMEOTUK network as a critical friend, is starting to think of strategies to tackle institutional racism, and now other newly formed UK occupational therapy affinity groups are doing the same.

The education sector appears to have fallen behind when dealing with the injustices, inequalities and inequities faced by minoritised people. This can be evidenced when looking at degree results of students from Black, Asian and minoritised backgrounds as opposed to their white counterparts (Universities UK and National Union of Students 2019). Time and time again in the UK, studies show on average that white students are more likely to leave university with a first- or upper-second-class degree as opposed to students from Black and minoritised backgrounds (Universities UK and National Union of Students 2019). Research confirms that the experiences we have as students have a huge impact on who we are likely to become as therapists (Richards & Galvaan 2018; Hammond *et al.* 2019). If we are exposed to the reality of the injustices individuals and communities face and can see or have experienced this first-hand, we may have even more drive to improve things moving forward. We must be open to having those difficult conversations and to critically reflecting on the inequity of our practice and previous experiences which may have contributed to the structural issues in the systems in which we are working or living. Studies demonstrate that it is imperative that abiding policies are formed which provide equitable chances for all, regardless of heritage or socio-economic background (Richards & Galvaan 2018; Hammond *et al.* 2019). These policies must address the institutionalised racism that we see across the world in various environments and sectors and in the profession of occupational therapy. Only by doing this will we then be able to work towards reducing the injustices and barriers that service users and communities face.

If the past few years have shown us anything, it is that we need to show learning from previous mistakes through impactful actions. We need to look at the racial inequalities and injustices across the board, see the effects these have in our profession and the wider population, and work towards making things more equitable for students, staff and service users alike (Thomas 2020).

AUTHOR'S VOICE: SIHLE

In co-writing this chapter, I am reminded of how I am affected by the consequences of racism and health inequalities/inequities. As a Black woman of African background, I find myself feeling unsure and insecure of my present and future for my family and my position in my career. Will I get gaslighted as aggressive and unapproachable if I speak the truth about racism and discrimination? Will it disrupt my career progression? Will it disenable me from receiving the right care if I need medical intervention? Will it stop my future child from being a statistic of police brutality? As a Black woman and an occupational therapist, I will continue the struggle to make things right through actions, no matter how small. We are only at the surface to try and disrupt racism and health inequities; we need to gather a growing collective to collaborate in this work within the profession, to show visible active allyship with our Black Asian and minoritised peers and service users.

AUTHOR'S VOICE: KOSIWA

Developing the content for this chapter has been a highly emotional journey. In all honesty, it has reminded me just how far we have yet to go and how much change is needed in society. Throughout my daily life, I am aware of this as a result of the nuanced racism I face as a young Black woman and a young Black occupational therapist. However, researching the topic and seeing it there in written form has been a truly humbling experience.

I hope and pray that better days are to come, for myself, my family, friends and wider community. However, we need to do more than hope and pray. We need committed and sustainable action and change to make a better life and future for us and those ahead of us. No one should be indifferent and inactive to the injustice, inequity and racism others face. There is no human excuse.

Conclusion

For transformative change to happen we must first recognise the issues as only then can the process of change start. It's not enough to just be not racist, as we must be antiracist (Kendi 2017). Occupational therapy as a practice is about transformation, about change for individuals and communities, so we should be applying our principles and skills to disrupt institutional racism in the profession and health and social care. As an occupational therapy profession, we have a long way to go and we must start by acknowledging the presence of institutional racism in the profession, before changing through both a top-down and bottom-up approach, as antiracism is everyone's responsibility. Our governments must start putting in place long-term strategies to address the systemic issues at hand, but the first step comes from us as individuals. We are accountable to ourselves, our peers and service users and must educate ourselves on issues of oppression, racism and inequities before we can form counter interventions to improve the day-to-day lives of service users and communities collaboratively.

To truly move forward, we must work together to keep issues like this at the forefront, to make change actions to disrupt the status quo of racism and health inequities as only then will we start to chip away sustainably at its systemic roots. It is the responsibility of each one of us to seek and implement change. Think of it like this: if we cannot all sit at the table to eat at the table, then we must remove the food from that table and make conditions where everyone can reach the food and thrive.

Reflective quadrant: Identifying, recording and understanding learning from the chapter

What? (Describe what have I learnt)	**Relevance?** (Why is this topic relevant to me/to my practice?) Relate/align to/with, e.g., research literature, professional bodies' proficiencies/competencies, service delivery/service user benefit, legislation – briefly and critically discuss)
How will this learning change me/my practice?	**What actions do I have to follow up on to develop my learning in this area or apply to my practice?** (SMART goal format or similar)

CHAPTER 2

Introduction to Critical Race Theory

Lily Owens and Shahedah Vawda

'Strange Fruit' became a protest song against horrific public lynching practices involving mostly Black Americans in the United States – practices that lasted until 1968 (National Association for the Advancement of Colored People 2022). A lynching is a 'public spectacle' that conveys a message to minoritized 'others' – one such message being 'that the law cannot protect [them]' (Taseer in Williams & Romer 2020). However, many argue that lynchings are still ongoing in their literal form and in new forms, for example school to prison pipeline, police murders (Campbell 2019; Pilkington 2021). A modern-day lynching was televised in 2020, with the public murder of George Floyd on an ordinary American street. This was a murder in which a Black family man was subjected to having the knee of a white police officer forcefully and relentlessly on his neck, taking his life. George Floyd's haunting words, 'I can't breathe', are a final testament of the devastating injustice by a representative of the 'system' and ultimately a reminder of how Black communities, in particular, continue to be stripped of their humanity and therefore, the right to justice, to this very day (The Guardian 2021).

This chapter introduces the reader to the concept of critical race theory and its relevance to occupational therapy. The chapter content answers three questions:

- What is critical race theory?
- How has white privilege and power influenced the direction of occupational therapy?
- How can critical race theory frame and actively contribute to antiracism agendas in theory and practice?

Historically, critical race theory (CRT) was born out of a life and death struggle for equal rights and justice in the United States, in a context of deep segregation and racism, often sanctioned and legitimized by the law itself. The draconian Jim Crow laws in the United States are a haunting example of how the law was pivotal in its systematic discrimination against Black people, responsible for racial segregation, the denial of the right to vote, and a refusal of basic rights such as secure, decent jobs, education and housing.

Rooted in critical legal scholarship, CRT sought to expose and redress racial injustices in the American legal system and American society more widely (Crenshaw et al. 1995). Its founding members were legal scholars, lawyers and activists (see for example Bell 1973, 1987; Crenshaw 1988, Delgado & Stefancic 2017; Matsuda et al. 1993 and others) who sought to highlight and challenge the systemic racial inequality they were witnessing and living in the United States. While Crenshaw did introduce the term intersectionality, the concept dates much further back to the early 1900s with Black feminists and voting rights (Hills Collins & Bilge 2020).

CRT centres on beliefs that racism is systemically normalised, meaning societal laws and rules are designed to uphold and continue racial injustices (Delgado & Stefancic 2017) and that this status quo must be recognized, so that it can be disrupted and challenged (Crenshaw 1988; 1997; Crenshaw et al. 1995; Delgado & Stefancic 2017). To support such recognition, CRT fundamentally allows for critical questioning of the 'very foundation of the liberal order – equality theory; legal reasoning, enlightenment rationalism and the neutrality of the principles of constitutional law' (Delgado & Stefancic 2017: 3), in which power is invested and reinforced. Essentially, CRT became a radical alternative lens to not only more conservative mainstream perspectives but also supposedly radical critical legal studies, which according to Black-American philosopher and Civil Rights activist Cornel West 'deconstructed liberalism, yet seldom addressed the role of deep-seated racism in American Life' (West 1995: xi).

In line with Bell's work, CRT fundamentally rejected dominant assertions that the law was one of neutrality, objectivity, colour-blindness and meritocracy, viewing such claims as 'camouflages for the self-interest of powerful entities of society' (Tate 1997: 235). Bell further coined the term 'interest-convergence', which argued that such powerful entities in society would only support racial advances when challenged, if it benefitted in some way those already in power or privileged positions (Bell 1980). Furthermore, CRT fundamentally challenged ahistoricism, insisting on contextual historical scrutiny of the law and an active recognition of the lived experiences of people of colour (Tate 1997). Delgado termed this as a 'call to context', highlighting the importance of context and the lived experiences of minoritized groups as a challenge against the dominant rhetoric of colour-blindness (Delgado & Stefancic 2017).

CRT also recognises the intersectional nature of oppressions, how various additional identities coming together (i.e. class, gender) can further uniquely shape racial injustices experienced (Crenshaw 1989). As such, '...an intersectional approach goes beyond conventional analysis... to 1) analyse social problems more fully; 2) shape more effective interventions; and 3) promote more inclusive coalitional advocacy' (African American Policy Forum 2009: 3).

While it is difficult to condense CRT into a chapter, Professor Gillborn provides a helpful conceptual map of key elements (see Box 2.1).

Box 2.1: CRT – a conceptual map (adapted from Gillborn 2007: 12)

Elements that define CRT

- Racism is endemic...'normal' not aberrant nor rare: deeply engrained legally and culturally.

- Crosses epistemological boundaries.

- Critique of civil rights laws as fundamentally limited.

- Critique of liberalism – claims of neutrality, objectivity, colour-blindness and meritocracy as camouflages.

- Call to context – challenges ahistoricism and recognizes experiential knowledge of people of colour, challenges systemic white supremacy and highlights the change of whiteness as racial identity to racialised forms of property and property rights that privilege whiteness.

Conceptual tools

- Storytelling and counter-stories.

- Interest convergence.
- Critical white studies.

CRT helps us to understand why it was predictable that in 2020/21 minoritized communities were disproportionately affected by the COVID-19 pandemic, despite many previously well-documented correlations between the social determinants of health and health outcomes (Marmot & Wilkinson 2005; Marmot *et al.* 2020b). This point was emphasised by Cornel West, who stated that George Floyd's 'public lynching' connected with the pandemic, pulling the 'cover off who we really are and what our system really is' (Muir 2020).

Practically, for minoritized practitioners like the authors of this chapter, CRT as a critical lens opens up avenues to explore how racism operates in systems such as education and healthcare (see for example Ladson-Billings 1998). Furthermore, CRT, with its focus on unmasking racism in the everyday and its accompanying emphasis on 'counter-narratives', gives people of colour and their struggle legitimacy by actively resisting narratives of the majority and making space for counter-voices to be centred and heard (Delgado & Stefancic 2017; Solorzano & Yosso 2001).

Routine critical practice incident and sense-making

We thought it would be helpful to begin this critical reflection by presenting the experience of a single critical incident at work from one of the authors of this chapter (S. Vawda) to consider and demonstrate the application of CRT's use of counter-narratives. This process can not only affirm the sense-making process for therapists of colour, but also contextualise such experiences in broader structural terms (Solorzano & Yosso 2001).

The presentation of these experiences should be read as a critical incident because these situations are personally troubling and traumatic, often requiring an ongoing process of sense-making (Sue *et al.* 2007a).

CRITICAL INCIDENT AND SENSE-MAKING – S. VAWDA

I am a South Asian woman of South African heritage. I have worked within inner London for the last 15 years as a community neuro-re-habilitation therapist. Given the demographic, my work has entailed navigating wide-ranging attitudes and political bearings within different communities. I have developed a thick skin.

This narrative involves a gentleman in his mid-sixties who had had a stroke. He had lived in one area for the last 50 years with his wife, family and friends nearby. Before our first home visit, I was aware of the resentment that some of the white community in this area had felt as they witnessed the change or 'loss' of their neighbourhood to various communities from different cultures.

On my first visit I was accompanied by my colleague, a person of Sri Lankan heritage. The patient's wife answered the door and we introduced ourselves, stating our roles, in response to which she asked when the therapist would be coming. I again explained that I was the occupational therapist and that the physiotherapist would be joining us later, acknowledging that it could be confusing as there were many professionals involved. We proceeded to meet the patient who was lying in bed in what appeared to be some pain. He seemed displeased to see us, stating that he had just been discharged the day before and had had a 'bad night'.

My role as a Band 7 occupational therapist in the team was to support people post-discharge, following up on whether they had appropriate equipment and services to start rehabilitation at home. The first session can be challenging as you try to establish a relationship of mutual trust within a brief timeframe. I understood within the first few minutes of meeting him that establishing a rapport would indeed be challenging, as he was in pain and not keen to participate and unwilling to attempt any functional movement. However, after 45 minutes my colleague and I had managed to persuade him to sit up in bed and facilitated a grooming session in bed, all while assessing his needs, providing education and reassurance.

As our session was drawing to a close, my Band 7 white male phys-iotherapist colleague arrived and openly expressed surprise that the patient had not been washed and dressed and demanded to know what we had achieved in our session – all in the presence of the patient and his wife. I attempted to explain that the patient had not been keen due to pain and that I would return in two days, as our colleague would be seeing him in the interim. However, I was interrupted by him stating that this outcome and my clinical reasoning were unacceptable, and it would put the patient at risk. He concluded with saying that he would have to discuss my performance with my manager. When I asked to address the matter outside, he refused to discuss it further. I excused myself from the session, ensuring that the patient and wife were aware that they would be seen by my colleague, and left rather shocked and shaken, not quite knowing how to comprehend what had happened.

An hour later I called my manager, who patiently listened to my description of what had transpired. For the sake of context, it is worth noting that this was not the first difficult encounter between me and my physiotherapist colleague, as we had previously differed in our management styles. As a senior therapist in my forties, I was determined to be professional and not let our differences affect the team dynamic, although it had started to become a source of personal anxiety. I had chosen not to openly confront him previously as I had assumed that I could manage our differences, despite him being seen as challenging to work with by others in the team. Following the visit, I knew that I had grounds to start a formal disciplinary investigation into his conduct, but I did not want to expend energy on a long stressful lawful process.

To summarise, my manager offered me a reconciliatory process with my physiotherapist colleague (as unbeknown to me at the time it was not the first time he had complained about me). I declined this intervention, as I did not wish to subject myself to further stress and as I did not feel equally culpable for the situation. My manager then met with us separately and I was offered her support by way of joining a mentorship scheme, and asked how best I would like to manage the situation. I stated that it needed to be made clear to him that his behaviour towards me as a colleague was unacceptable, that I would explore the mentorship scheme, and that I would reflect further on what action was relevant.

Thereafter I was asked to present an in-service session to our team with another white female team colleague regarding unconscious bias and racism. My manager's attempts to support me were well intentioned but not impactful; I still felt traumatised by the incident while having continually to confront my physiotherapist colleague at work.

Following this initial incident, on a subsequent home visit while awaiting my colleague, the patient's wife casually mentioned on three separate occasions how grubby my colleague's clothes were, and how he 'always smelt of curry'. To this I replied that he was always professional in his conduct and attire and was therefore well loved by colleagues and patients. After several such comments, I raised what I perceived to be prejudicial remarks to our team and asked what our team policy was before addressing it with the wife. I attempted to discuss how to raise it with the patient's wife but was told by some members of the team that I should not be so sensitive and that I needed to understand that the wife was of an older generation, especially as the comments made did not sound openly 'racist' and that she 'meant no harm'. However, when pushed, the team agreed that any further comments would be unacceptable. It was suggested that if I felt strongly about future comments, I should state that the team would not tolerate racial slurs. When I asked what the team policy was, I was directed to the NHS policy on antiracism.[1]

Sense-making is using counter-narrative to elucidate the hegemonic structures and contextualization of the therapist of colour's experience (Solorzano & Yosso 2001):

> 'Counter storytelling' and use of experiential knowledge by people of colour is central to CRT as a powerful tool with which to expose the devastating consequences of microaggression and disrupt the norm of racism. (Gillborn 2007; Cousins 2019)

Here are example narratives that could be seen to gaslight my experiences: perhaps my colleague just had a different therapeutic approach to mine; perhaps these were 'personality differences'; perhaps the wife didn't mean to be offensive, and I was being overly sensitive; perhaps my manager did not know the best way to deal with the situation and it was my role to support her. No one wants 'to play the race card', because it causes tension, emotion and feelings of coming into an unsafe space and more. The phrase 'to play the race card' is a power position to maintain the dominant gaslighting narrative.

How these issues were raised and dealt with one could argue was undoubtedly determined and driven by the powerful factors of

---

[1]   www.england.nhs.uk/london/2020/06/05/nhs-london-statement-on-racism

intersectionality – gender, religion, race, culture – and the invisibility of institutional whiteness. Individual actions cannot gain traction without the systems of power acknowledging that institutional racism and discrimination exist and divide employees into oppressed/subordinating vs. emboldened positionalities (Fanon 2004) and enable individuals to act aligned to their positionality accordingly.

Questions to explore

- Could it be that my white male physiotherapist colleague was emboldened institutionally to overrule my clinical reasoning and undermine my professional judgement in front of a patient and their family in an unprofessional and authoritarian way, as I am a brown Asian Muslim woman?

- How is the NHS policy on antiracism enabling the status quo of racism to remain?

- Why did my white male physiotherapist colleague think it acceptable to treat me, a brown Asian Muslim woman, as a subordinate, despite us being in the same professional band, and openly threaten to report me to higher management?

- As a white male colleague, did he feel he had to dominate and demonstrate a power play by having his final words unquestioned, given that I had tended to not directly challenge him before? Why did I not assertively disrupt his power play?

- Did the patient/family expect that a brown person could not be the authority figure, but that the ultimate authority would be that of the white male/person? Why did I not assertively disrupt this viewpoint?

- What effect did questioning my knowledge/skills have on my white patient and his family, who demonstrated they were embedded within the norm of whiteness?

- Did my public dressing down erode their trust in my clinical competence and set the context for future interactions?

- Why did my team of fellow health professionals fail to see the complexity of the situation, and fail to acknowledge the significance of the 'casual' racism towards my rehabilitation support worker?

- What processes were there within the service and the institution (NHS at large) to recognise and support antiracist practice?

- Were the offers of reconciliation and mentorship sufficient to address the unacknowledged structural racism that enabled this incident?

- Was I best placed to deliver team training given the highly charged nature of the event?

Counter-narrative reflections

To ask my team/service to deal with this incident would highlight the dilemma that DiAngelo (2018) describes as the good-bad binary – the belief that being a good person (post the abolishment of slavery) and complicity with racism are mutually exclusive. DiAngelo (2018) clarifies this as the dilemma of how a person could hold racist views if they are a good person. Bell (2009) argues that the superior white narrative may not materially but rather psychically advance the white working-class position by magnifying the white supremacy ideology.

Some of the team chose to think of the wife's comments as 'casually racist'. Everyday racism is emboldened institutionally by policies, practices, culture and leadership (Cousins 2019). However, as explained by antiracism campaigner Alexander Leon, the idea that some forms of racism are casual and therefore more acceptable than more blatant forms of racism fails to acknowledge that both are racism and cause suffering, and both are unacceptable. It also centres the intentions of the person perpetuating racism rather than centring the attention on the receiver of racism and the consequences of this behaviour, which is dehumanization and the outcomes of perpetual embodied trauma (Cousins 2019; Williams 2019). Other team members took the liberal-ist stance of not 'seeing colour', but this colour-blindness denies the everyday lived realities that those identities bring. This is a non-racist position that supports racism by taking a neutral position, instead of being antiracist, which is actively against all forms of racism and discrimination (Kendi 2019).

As occupational therapists, we are trained in understanding the interrelated dynamic equilibrium between the person, environment and occupation (PEO model). However, we acknowledge that the PEO model does not account for systemic patterns of exclusion. We are taught to analyse how the environment significantly impacts on the person's capacity to effectively partake (occupational performance) in activities they want and need to do (occupations). Knowing this, there is still the expectation that occupational therapists from Black, Asian and minoritised backgrounds should continue to work within an institutionally racist environment, without any support to adequately address the consequences of experiencing this everyday racism which affects them psychologically and physically, and impacts their career progression (Williams 2019; NHS England 2021). We therefore internalise normalised oppression, and it is 'literally killing us' says Professor Williams (2019). Through his 'Everyday Discrimination Scale' he has gathered evidence regarding how powerfully the little indignities affect our emotional and physical wellbeing; for example, increased inflammatory markers put one at risk for a broad range of issues, such as coronary heart disease, increased blood pressure, lower birth weight babies for expectant mothers, and, in adults, premature death (Williams 2019).

Unfortunately, the measures to remedy the situation through team education placed the burden of addressing racism in the team on me, the brown individual who experienced the racism. Derrick Bell (2009) coined the term 'contradictory story closure', which talks of these seemingly progressive measures that act as a safety valve to allow just the right amount of racism to be maintained (Gillborn 1998): 'too much would be destabilizing – the victims would rebel. Too little would forfeit important pecuniary and psychic advantages for those in power' (Delgado 1995: 80). Time and again people of colour are asked to tell their stories of grief and trauma, 'trauma porn', to inspire change, but apart from assuaging white guilt, little changes structurally. The manager should have shown leadership and organised the actions, turning to policies and resources and identifying how racism would be documented and dealt with. The manager in the power position should be doing the work and role-modelling allyship and antiracist behaviour.

As structural racism and discrimination remain unacknowledged it perpetuates a level of colour-blindness based on the assumption that the NHS is an equitable service which treats all its patients and staff justly. This means that the NHS antiracism policy is not effective for the workplace. According to CRT, this means that only the most glaring and 'easy' forms of discrimination are addressed as lesser incidents (Bell 2009). It was a lost opportunity to question how the service could have provided adequate support and could begin to practise in an antiracist way. To acknowledge racism, resist it and work in a different framework is seen as 'wrong' as it defies this norm, according to CRT. Racist stereotypes play out unless we consciously set out to stop them (Williams 2019). Indeed, what is arguably required, at the very least, is a deeper acknowledgement of the reality of racism in everyday experiences for people of colour, which does not stop when we become therapists and educators, and the psychological traumas this may inevitably entail, alongside wider structural recognition of its systemic operation (Picower 2009).

CRT offers a critical lens which is necessary to understand the reality and work on disruption through impactful changes.

Sadly, sense-making processes of trauma may take years, while many NHS organisations are still not wanting to acknowledge institutional racism, despite sufficient data to validate this (Public Health England 2020c; NHS England 2021). If the sense-making process is not carried out with due care it is capable of re-traumatising the individual, long after critical incidents have occurred. CRT values and validates such sense-making and narratives as counter-narratives, while Freire (1972: 26) recognised that the best individuals to understand the 'terrible significance of an oppressive society' are the 'oppressed themselves'.

CRT has been criticised in the UK and United States, mostly by conservative/republican quarters, and accused of peddling socialist ideologies and centring race as a major focus with societally disruptive consequences (see for example Warmington 2019 and Bell 2009 to help understand some of these issues). CRT is a theory that can be debated and discussed just like any other; it is a critical lens, but not the only lens. It is suggested that those who object should propose an alternate lens to critique racism and its many negative impacts.

What is CRT doing in a 'nice' field like occupational therapy?

It is increasingly being argued with urgency that occupational therapy is implicit in systematic racist operations (Kronenberg 2020b; Ramugondo 2020), peddling white supremacy (Grenier 2020), inherently centred on Eurocentric knowledge (Arday *et al.* 2020) and the normalisation of whiteness as the way to be and do, while 'othering' those who do not fit such ideas of normalcy in theory and practice (Hammell 2021, 2009; Owens 2016).

Furthermore, there is an increased focus on action, including calls for the adoption of antiracist occupational therapy practices (Farias & Simaan 2020), antiracist education (Arday *et al.* 2020), the decolonising of the curriculum (Simaan 2020b), and recognition of the ways the occupation itself has contributed to 'systemic racism against Black people in the United States' (Lavalley & Robinson Johnson 2022: 1). Such calls appear paradoxical, considering that occupational therapy purports to be a profession built on the principles of social justice, person-centredness, social inclusion and holism (Hocking 2017), calling for its therapists to be 'change agents' tasked with the implementation of these in practice in the communities in which they work (Finlayson 2013). However, as indicated in other chapters, transformation for antiracism in the profession needs engagement from collaborative collectives for momentum.

CRT offers a radical alternative lens, a lens that differs from the 'taken for granted' lenses that we wear every day (Milner 2006). Epistemologically and ontologically, this is important, because the sole focus on the individual without the context of powerful structures is not normalised in CRT. Instead, it is assumed, as with critical theories, that individuals are not free but involved in immense power struggles, impacting on what people of colour are genuinely able to be and do. In CRT, such power struggles centre on race as a powerful social construct and weapon, systematically dehumanising minoritised 'others' to justify the subjugation and violation of minoritized individuals and communities. Ideology is important here, because it – in this case 'whiteness' (see Grenier 2020 for a meaningful discussion on this) – is so deeply engrained ontologically and epistemologically that it is taken for granted and invisible (McIntosh 1989) to those who not only hold power but action such power on 'others' in theory and practice.

CRT, then, acts as a lens that focuses on that racialized violence by pulling such violence out from the margins, centring it and thereby demonstrating the terrible significance of a racist social system on the 'other' (Delgado & Stefancic 2017).

Occupational therapy, with its well-meaning idealism, is not immune to complicity, as it does not sit in a social vacuum, but is inextricably involved in a powerful political, social and economic system (Foucault 1970) that reinforces ideological values of whiteness and white supremacy. So, when profession-specific statements express solidarity with the oppressed, without the context of oppression and, more specifically, without taking responsibility for the profession's own involvement in oppression, such 'solidarity' positioning is arguably an act that Freire would have referred to as 'false generosity' (Smith 2010: 134). Dr Kronenberg argued such a point eloquently, following an invitation to respond to the *Journal of Occupational Science*'s position statement on racism specifically (Kronenberg 2021a: 400), calling for one's 'gaze [on racism] to be turned inwardly', to critically 'interrogat[e] how this oppressive mechanism may manifest in its [own] operations'. He further questioned, among other valuable points, the failure to interrogate, essentially the ongoing perpetuation of an 'apolitical and ahistorical... whiteness-based approach' to studying occupation, in line with CRT's fundamental challenges to ahistoricism.

And therein lies a fundamental problem to making occupational therapy capable of genuine interrogation of racism in its own backyard – the avoidance to date, by the profession, to admit (and to consequently start to make attempts to dismantle) its own complicity in racist operations, and therefore its own complicity in injustices and health inequalities in this present day, demonstrating an apolitical and ahistorical stance regarding its colonialist roots. After all, as Guajardo *et al.* (2015: 4) importantly pointed out, 'it is impossible to escape the political and ethical implications of our actions'. What is required, then, is the start of a process which sees the profession grappling with its own complicities of racism and misuses of power, actively acknowledging historical, political and structural processes, from a much-needed positioning of humility, critical self-interrogation and transparency.

Racism, specifically, is the state-sanctioned or extra-legal production and exploitation of group-differentiated vulnerability to premature death. (Gilmore 2007: 247)

The extent and direct consequences of health inequalities have been starkly exposed by the COVID-19 pandemic, with people of colour dying disproportionally in the UK and internationally (Devakumar *et al.* 2020). Racism is now considered a public health crisis (Acosta 2020) – one that we can no longer ignore (Devakumar *et al.* 2020).

It can be argued that occupational therapy, by way of its own complicity in racist operations, is contributing to health inequalities. Furthermore, a dangerous lack of critical self-interrogation (Kronenberg 2021a) is arguably creating conditions in which racism as a structural force of power is able to thrive unnoticed and unquestioned, impacting detrimentally on minoritized 'othered' individuals and their communities. These include its own students, therapists and educators (see, for example, BAMEOTUK YouTube channel podcasts; Simaan 2020b; Guajardo Córdoba 2020). Symptoms (not exhaustive) of such conditions entail:

- Many students, educators and therapists from minoritized communities not feeling as though they entirely belong to the profession (Owens 2016).

- Well-meaning therapists misunderstanding mistrust from minoritized client communities in practice as deficit without understanding the permanence of racism (Fernando 2017).

- The primacy of western models and theories of knowing and being reinforcing whiteness and Eurocentric westernized ideals, including the cult of the individual (Kantartzis & Molineux 2011; Laliberte Rudman 2013).

- Systematic un-acknowledging of whiteness in the curriculum (Arday *et al.* 2020) and more.

- Making efforts to widen participation by trying to attract minoritized students (in an effort to create a more 'diverse' workforce to counter health inequalities) without directly addressing racism as a fundamental driver of such health inequalities, in which the profession itself, is complicit.

- Trying to recruit 'diverse' students without explicit commitment to their health and wellbeing once recruited, inclusive of a recognition of continued high drop-out rates, a curriculum and theories that do not reflect 'them' (Hammell 2013) and potential university and practice placement encounters of racism and discrimination, likely to cause further psychological harm (Thomas 2020; Fernando 2017).

Conclusion

Critically turning the lens on the profession in order to build 'antiracist' conditions in occupational therapy appears fundamentally important (see, for example, Hammell 2011; Sakellariou & Pollard 2017; Laliberte Rudman 2014; Thomas 2020; Ramugondo & Kronenberg 2015; Guarjado Córdoba 2020; Malfitano *et al.* 2014).

Such a critical inward gaze is arguably a radical political act of discomfort, and even as Nicholls and Elliot (2019) suggest, mourning. Essentially, such action could contribute to disrupting and dismantling the master's house (of whiteness) as proposed by Audre Lorde (1994) and adopted more widely across student-led activism initiatives outside occupational therapy (see, for example, Tehrani 2015).

The road is not an easy one, nor is the discomfort caused by the putting on of critical lenses necessarily always bearable, particularly for those who have naturally held power for so long. Toni Morrison painfully alludes to a potential existential crisis, by saying that when: 'you can only be tall because someone else is on their knees, then you have a serious problem' (Toni Morrison Interview with Charlie Rose (PBS 1993}).

Ultimately, though, employing critically radical lenses to enable a sense-making and deconstruction process, which helps to challenge inequalities, does not have to result in hopelessness (Gillborn 2011). Instead, it is arguably necessary to deconstruct in order to begin the process of building back fairer (Marmot *et al.* 2020a). Importantly, such criticality is not a one-off event, but a lifelong disposition of becoming and remaining critically conscious and thereby ethically and authentically committed to the people (Adorno 1978).

Reflective quadrant: Identifying, recording and understanding learning from the chapter

What? (Describe what have I learnt)

Relevance? (Why is this topic relevant to me/to my practice? Relate/align to/with, e.g., research literature, professional bodies' proficiencies/competencies, service delivery/service user benefit, legislation – briefly and critically discuss)

How will this learning change me/my practice?

What actions do I have to follow up on to develop my learning in this area or apply to my practice? (SMART goal format or similar)

Contribution of Racism in Racial Inequalities, Health Inequities and Social Determinants of Health and Occupational Therapy

Kalimah Ibrahiim, Kwaku Agyemang, Fasloen Adams

Introduction

This chapter aims to explore and understand the factors contributing to racial and health inequalities and inequities and the role occupational therapy has in working towards addressing this with minoritised populations. There is an emphasis on the social determinants of health in this chapter, but we want to remind the reader that the determinants of health are wider than this; there are political, structural, historical and intergenerational determinants of health and more, and we encourage the reader to explore these too. The words of R.H. Tawney (1931: 57) (a white English man, an economic historian and ethical socialist) sit well in the introduction to the chapter:

> It is the mark of a civilized society to aim at eliminating such inequalities as have their source, not in individual differences, but in its own organisation, and that individual differences, which are a source of social energy, are more likely to ripen and find expression if social inequalities are, as far as practicable, diminished.

Tawney was elucidating that inequalities are created by people, organisations and structures, and people are in organisations and are the ones that create structures. Hence people can change the circumstances to reduce or remove the impacts of this socially constructed situation.

The chapter content covers three critical questions:

- What are some of the health inequalities and inequities experienced by racially minoritized populations?

- What factors maintain racial inequalities in society?

- What is the role of occupational therapy in addressing health inequities?

Background

There are health disparities among different minoritised ethnicities and marginalised/socio-economically disadvantaged groups in the UK and globally. According to Marmot *et al.* (2020a) this gap is widening and has not reduced since 2010 due to chronic underfunding to effectively address the social determinants of health as a priority, which Marmot puts down to systemic racism and discrimination. The social determinants of health are the fundamental circumstances that influence our health outcomes and have a pivotal role in our life expectancy. They include, but are not limited to, three main factors: a person's socio-economic environment, a person's physical environment, and a person's individual behaviours, education and beliefs. The conditions in which we are born, grow, live, work and age all influence our overall health outcomes, wellbeing and life expectancy (Marmot *et al.* 2020a). The World Health Organisation (WHO 2022) defines health as not just the absence of ill-health but the combination of the physical health, mental wellbeing and social dimensions, including the number of years a person is living healthily.

Even before birth, these determinants have an impact on our lives. The family we are born into, access to good quality maternity services, access to good healthcare, adequate housing, lifestyle, good food, good quality education, social capital, secure jobs, money, reduced stress, civic engagement and power, all collectively determine our health outcomes (Woodall *et al.* 2015; WHO 2021). Although occupation is not listed as a social determinant of health, we would suggest that it should be, because occupation – that is, participation in meaningful activity/ies – has an influence on health and wellbeing and hence the ability to thrive.

One stark example of a health disparity can be found in maternal health. The disparities in maternal healthcare between those from a Black and minoritised background and their white counterparts have been well documented. A report by the National Perinatal Epidemiology Unit and University of Oxford (2021) found that in the UK, Black women were almost five times more likely, and Asian women nearly twice as likely, to die in pregnancy and childbirth when compared to their white counterparts. Another data set from the Department of Health (NHS Digital 2022) shows that Black people are five times more likely to be detained under the Mental Health Act and ten times more likely to be given a community treatment order than their white counterparts.

The data trends are showing that Black people are discriminated against not only in the health system but also in the justice system. According to the UK Home Office, Black people are more likely to be stopped and searched by the police than their white counterparts. From April 2019 to March 2020 there were 211 documented stop and searches by police on Black/Black other per 1000 Black people in England and Wales compared to 6 in 1000 white people (Home Office 2021). This kind of structural racism and discrimination has been shown to lead to poor health outcomes (Gee & Ford 2011; Williams 2016). There appears to be a link between the inequities in the health and justice system for Black and minoritised populations. For example, Black populations in Britain are more likely to be detained under the Mental Health Act (Davies 2022), although the Lammy (2017) review identified that on arriving at prison, Black and minoritised individuals are less likely to have mental health concerns compared to their white peers. The chronic under investment in mental health services has led to Black people 'with mental illnesses [having] encountered increased engagement with the carceral system' (Jordan *et al.* 2021: 9). Systemic racism and racial inequity are visible throughout systems whether it be health and social care, education or justice. The data evidence states that health disparities affecting minoritised communities living in western countries are not due to genetic health differences but are a result of health inequities caused by systemic racism, that are a function of the historical and present unequal distribution of social, economic and environmental resources (Marmot *et al.* 2020a). Marmot *et al.* (2020a) also say that the underfunded areas have a high population of minoritised and marginalised populations, hence systemic racism and discrimination play a main role in this chronic lack of investment.

The coronavirus pandemic highlighted the presence of racial inequalities and health inequities. Racially minoritised and marginalised groups were found to be more likely to become infected with the virus and more likely to become seriously ill and die from it. Factors such as occupations and access to healthcare services among these groups have been said to be some of the main contributors to this (Public Health England 2020b). These caring and elementary roles were some of the most needed during the pandemic and could not be achieved while working from home. With racially minoritised and marginalised groups often living in multi-generational households, having to travel on public transport as well as having jobs that engage them with the public not only exposes them to the virus, but also their entire households. They did not have the scaffolding around them to protect them from ill-health and death during this time period, and this was due to institutional racism; the policies, practices and work culture were stacked against these populations (Public Health England 2020b).

Social capital is the presence or absence of resources and networks available in a community. Hahn *et al.* (2018) suggest that to address the social determinants of health there needs to be a place-based solution – addressing the environments where people live will improve health outcomes (NHS England 2020). Social capital is not necessarily a geographic area but the access an individual or family has to a society that enables them and their community to function effectively or not. Social capital includes tangible assets such as access to safe public spaces, property, good quality housing, money, transport, and intangible assets such as social class, people, interpersonal relationships, access to knowledge, trust and power (Woodall *et al.* 2015). For example, if you are born into a family with wealth and power (with tangible and intangible assets) your social determinants of health will be more favourable. This may mean that a person will have access to good healthcare, good food, good quality education, good quality jobs, good social capital, have good health outcomes and be less likely to live in a state of poverty or hardship. If you are born into a family without tangible assets, you may have poor quality housing, a lack of access to safe green spaces, unsafe public areas, homelessness, poor quality education, low paid jobs. Without intangible assets you may experience poverty, poor interpersonal relationships, low educational attainment, limited or no access to knowledge, lack of trust and power, and you could have poor health outcomes in adulthood (Woodall *et al.* 2015). Moreover, social support and social inclusion are protective factors against ill-health, and therefore social exclusion and isolation contribute to poorer health outcomes. The child is advantaged or disadvantaged depending on the circumstances they are born into (Woodall *et al.* 2015). The majority in the category of not having tangible assets are the minoritised and marginalised communities, so there are systemic issues, such as leadership, culture, policies, practices and processes enabling this to occur as business as usual.

The World Health Organisation (2021) classifies early childhood development as a social determinant of health, therefore our early experiences in childhood can shape our lives as we grow positively or negatively. Adverse childhood experiences (ACEs) are traumatic stressful experiences that children are exposed to. These can be an isolated event or prolonged events such as domestic violence, sexual abuse, poverty, poor education, crime, trauma, their environment, homelessness, substance misuse (illicit drugs and excessive alcohol consumption), poor mental health, lack of trust, low economic status, food poverty and war to name a few (Golden 2021). A growing number of studies are showing that ACEs scores differ by heritage backgrounds, with greater impact on Black and Latinx people (Sacks & Murphey 2018). Any threat to a child's safety and security can impact on their worldview and willingness to engage with wider society. Research suggests that the more ACEs a child has, the greater their risk of issues in adulthood, such as heart disease, cancer, chronic stress, mental ill-health, premature death, substance misuse, violence, becoming a victim of violence, entering the criminal justice system, low productivity and other problems (Bellis *et al.* 2013; Chang *et al.* 2019). ACEs can have a generational impact, where their children then experience ACEs and the issues then have debilitating effects across more than one lifespan. The UK National ACE study reported that 47 per cent of adults experienced at least one ACE in childhood and 9 per cent of the UK population have four or more ACEs (Bellis *et al.* 2013). This is a significant number of adults who will have poor health outcomes in the UK. However, ACEs could be reduced by addressing the social determinants of health, investing in prevention and early intervention and narrowing the inequalities gap. This will also have an impact on generations to come and improve health outcomes (Center on the Developing Child 2021).

Racially minoritised and marginalised groups are likely to experience inequities due to living in deprivation, limited access to green spaces, poor access to safe and secure housing, inconsistent access to and experience of health services, living in areas of high rates of crime and violence, high unemployment rates – all caused primarily by political will to perpetually under-fund and under-resource public and welfare services (Marmot *et al.* 2020a). These experiences could also lead to some members of these communities experiencing psychosocial distress. The dyadic relationship between experiences of psychosocial distress/social exclusion and the systemic barriers such as institutional racism compounds the effects of health inequities (Marmot *et al.* 2020a). Marmot *et al.* (2020a) purport that to reduce the widening gap in health equity you need money, and this is doable with political willingness. This means investment in the early years of life, starting with maternal health, through to providing people with living wages, with affordable housing and access to nutritious foods (Marmot *et al.* 2020a). Living in a perpetual environmental state of inequity has long-term negative impacts on people's wellbeing, educational progress and ability to thrive, thus widening the health gap further (Thomas 2022).

Before Marmot's first report on reducing health inequality, published in 2010, there was already a focus on social determinants and systemic racism in the 1968 Kerner Commissioned Report (Kerner Commission 1968) and the book, *Unequal Treatment*, by Smedley *et al.* (2003) in the United States. Both these identified that systemic racism is causing the continued unequal access to health and social care, inequity in service provision for minoritised and marginalised groups, and therefore health disparities, poverty, ghettos and lack of access and opportunities to thrive as individuals and communities. Furthermore, the Kerner Commission reported that the discrimination faced by the Black and Latinx communities was constructed and maintained by America's white society and institutions, and warned that it would create a two-tier unequal hierarchical society, where the white population would continue to benefit by keeping the Black population disadvantaged (George 2018).

The potential role of occupational science and occupational therapy in addressing systemic racism

Jungersen's (1992) article 'Culture, theory and the practice of occupational therapy in New Zealand/Aotearoa' lays out that occupational therapy needs cultural integration and political awareness explicitly incorporated into practice through occupational therapy models to address the social issues caused by racism. Continuing that, there is a need to change occupational therapy models of practice away from being ethnically neutral or western centric in their make-up (Jungersen 1992). McConnell (2022) follows on from this and identifies the use of the Racially Informed Care (RIC) practice model in occupational therapy to enable Black, Indigenous, People of Color (BIPOC) persons to cope with racism and thrive in their lives. Occupational science is a cognate discipline to occupational therapy, in that it informs occupational therapy through the studying of how and why people do their everyday activities (occupations) in alignment with human rights and hence occupational justice. Occupational justice is 'the right of every individual to be able to meet basic needs and to have equal opportunities and life chances to reach toward [their] potential but specific to the individual's engagement in diverse and meaningful occupation' (Wilcock & Townsend 2009: 193). As occupational therapists, if we are concerned about people's ability to carry out their occupations, we must work on understanding the factors that will impact on planned treatment/interventions, such as racism. Occupational therapy training includes understanding the dynamic interrelationship of the environment and the person's abilities to participate in activities they need and want to do (occupations) (Duncan 2020). Inequity in access to health and social care services is widely documented and, due to institutional racism (Charasse-Pouélé & Fournier 2006; Gardiner *et al.* 2021; Chan *et al.* 2020), is an occupational justice concern because structural racism and discrimination are creating inequities in lived experiences resulting in reduced life expectancies, poor health outcomes, quality of life and living standards.

Although within occupational therapy, health disparities, racism and ethnicity are not unfamiliar topics (Rudman *et al.* 2018; Braveman & Bass-Haugen 2009; Bass-Haugen 2009), many argue that the profession needs to play an active role in reducing the disparities in healthcare. In 2006, Watson highlighted that occupational therapists should aim to assist people who are disadvantaged or disempowered by creating empowering and enabling opportunities (Watson 2006). In addition, Nelson (2007) cautioned that failure to consider the imbalances of power and privilege in the different world contexts would lead to these issues not being addressed and would disempower people. In the World Federation of Occupational Therapists' (WFOT) (2020: 1) statement on systemic racism, members are reminded of their responsibility to bring about change through advocacy and that it is essential that occupational therapy practitioners 'address the systematic discrimination, oppression, and injustice that are pervasive in health and social care services around the world'. Occupation contributes to social determinants of health, and meaningful and valued activities that help the person and communities thrive are a human right, and hence have a positive impact on a person's health outcomes. Occupational therapists need to be aware of the racism and social injustices, to enable them to understand their service user groups' needs. The WFOT (2020) further urges members to focus their action on ensuring improved equity and justice around the social determinants of health by disrupting the outcomes from societal dynamics, including racism, poverty, discrimination and oppressive systems. The WFOT has been around since the 1950s and has made its intentions known about its antiracism 'wishes' (WFOT 2020) but following through with impactful actions has been limited. Although there appears to be a recognition and acknowledgement that occupational therapists need to be working in this realm, perhaps the limited explicit direction from the WFOT to include antiracism, history of colonialism and more topics in curricula, impacts the knowledge and ability of occupational therapists to effectively work from a social justice approach explicitly and consistently.

The contextual systems of some health and social care services around the globe in which occupational therapists work also impact their ability to bring about social justice change. There are some occupational therapists re-addressing imbalance, for example the METUIA project at the University of São Paulo in Brazil. This is intended to enable communities to resist rights violations, systemic discrimination and oppression, to create conditions where communities can thrive collaboratively.[1] METUIA has worked with children where there have been high absences from schools by introducing community student leaders who are real models, and this has helped to reduce absences significantly (Malfitano et al. 2022).

Occupational therapists must usually fit the mould of the service, rather than being allowed to be innovative while working in a statutory service. Professional bodies around the globe should ensure that practical training on addressing systemic racism, discrimination and injustice

---

[1]   https://sites.usp.br/mestrado-profissional-terapiaocupacional/en/metuia

is a priority and should be one of the competencies therapists need to achieve. Occupational therapy and occupational science should aim to achieve a deeper understanding of the impact of health and social care inequalities and inequities, systemic racism and social determinants of health on a person's ability to participate in occupations of meaning and occupational performance to deliver authentic equitable practice, as areas of fundamental priority. Emery-Whittington (2021: 153) sums up with clarity that as a profession, 'Honest examination...alongside indigenous justice frameworks can advance critical praxes of...occupation and re-connect occupation with justice and equity'.

AUTHOR'S VOICE: FASLOEN – link between occupational opportunity and racial health inequity in South Africa

I was born and still live in South Africa, and I lived through the last two decades of Apartheid. Apartheid in South Africa is due to settler colonialism and was governed by various legal laws aimed at keeping different minoritized groups separated to their detriment and for the gain and advantage of the white populations. Apartheid is systemic racism and its legacies continue to negatively influence all social determinants of health, which in turn has a significant influence on the occupational choices of many minoritised and marginalised people within South Africa (McLean & McMillan 2009). There were many laws which governed the lives of the Black, brown, 'coloured' (a term used in South Africa to identify people of mixed heritage) and Indian people, including the Groups Areas Act of 1950, which forced different minoritised groups to live in different physical locations, and the Extension of University Education Act of 1959 which prevented Black, brown and Indian students from attending historically white universities (Gandhi-Luthuli Documentation Centre. UKZN, n.d.).

Apartheid laws forced the oppressed minoritised individuals and communities to engage in unfamiliar occupations and gave them limited engagement in familiar occupations, causing occupational alienation ('deep feelings of incompatibility with the occupations associated with a place, situation, or others to the extent that basic needs and wants appear impossible to attain or maintain' (Wilcock & Hocking 2015: 258)) and occupational deprivation ('points to externally imposed barriers to valued, meaningful occupations necessary for wellbeing' (Hocking 2017: 33)). Apartheid limited access to resources, occupational choices and freedom of association, to name just a few aspects. In essence, it impacted on the occupational justice and general health of the minoritised people. During Apartheid, access to health services was very fragmented and inequitably distributed among the four different minoritised groups (Maphumulo & Bhengu 2019) with more health resources available to white South Africans and the fewest resources allocated to Black South Africans. Apartheid legislating systemically racist systems of segregation is an example of occupational Apartheid, defined by Kronenberg as:

> the segregation of groups of people through the restriction or denial of access to dignified and meaningful participation in occupations of daily life on the basis of race, colour, disability, national origin, age, gender, sexual preference, religion, political beliefs, status in society, or other characteristics. (Kronenberg *et al.* 2015: 22)

The laws were used to legitimise racial capital and the acts of dehumanization, and occupationally restrict Black people to advantage white people.

Systemic racism is impacting the minoritised population's health and wellbeing in South Africa due to occupational Apartheid and occupational injustice causing a reduction in occupational choice, which in turn leads to disempowerment and decreases health and wellbeing. The associated inequitable distribution and allocation of funds for social determinants of health, including access to, for example, appropriate housing, education, access to adequate healthcare and food security, are caused by the legacy of occupational Apartheid which will live on for generations to come. More than ten years after Apartheid in South Africa, education levels are still the lowest among the Black populations, and for these groups poverty and unemployment remain high (Mariotti & Fourie 2014), thus continuing to decrease the social determinants of health for other generations. Similarly, access to adequate healthcare remains a challenge for the minoritised and marginalised communities due to remaining inequities in the allocation of resources and continuing poor quality of public healthcare services (Maphumulo & Bhengu 2019). Hence Kronenberg and colleagues questioned whether occupational therapy and occupational science, with their eyes on societal benefit and occupation justice, could be resources that enable society in South Africa to 'humanize and heal itself' (Kronenberg *et al.* 2015: 22).

Contribution of occupational therapy to health inequities and health disparities

There are many considerations we need to contemplate in discussing the contribution of occupational therapy to health inequities and health disparities. First, personal discrimination by healthcare providers was identified as a cause of health disparities, but it's not the only one. Institutional discrimination and systemic racism are as important as individual discrimination because they are often supported by institutional policies, practices and processes (Williams & Rucker 2000). Williams & Rucker (2000) over 20 years ago suggested that strategies needed to be implemented to eliminate racial inequities and should be made a priority to improve health outcomes for minoritised groups. These conversations have been going on for decades and, as the 2020 Marmot review stated, not much has improved; in fact, the disparities have widened (Marmot *et al.* 2020a).

Within occupational therapy, we need to acknowledge that the initial foundations of the profession were based on Western European and Northern American values (Iwama 2006). Owens (2016) argued that whiteness is entrenched in the profession's ontology and epistemology and this whiteness is invisible to many in the profession who have been taught to accept the traditional western-centric foundations. Consequently, most occupational therapy services focused more on an individualistic approach rather than a collective. Western ideologies focus on individualization and on the individual's needs. But in countries on the eastern/southern side of the continuum, for example South African, Caribbean, New Zealand and Asian cultures, occupational therapies value and support their collective traditions for the good of the individual, and community, and the families, extended families and wider communities assist the person by working collaboratively to facilitate and enable the individual to thrive. Decisions are made together with the person and the community to build a way forward for the person to transform the way they want and need to (Nkosi & Daniels 2007). It is only recently that the WFOT's definition of occupation changed to include activities performed by families and communities (WFOT

2010), while Ramugondo and Kronenberg in 2015 added that occupations are not always focused on individuals but also how community works together for collective wellbeing and for individual transformation. Thus, most models, theories and assessment and intervention modalities are focused on the individual and not on collectivism and the community population (Adams & Casteleijn 2014).

With the introduction of occupational science in the latter part of the 21st century, occupational scientists started unpacking the contextual impact on occupation, which includes racism (Adams & Casteleijn 2014), although still not discussing the history, for example the paradox that exists because the father of occupational science, Locke, had racist leanings (we are being diplomatic when using the latter term) (Emery-Whittington & Te Maro 2018). Similarly, in the mid and late 1990s there was an increased focus on multicultural awareness, as seen in literature; however, until recently the focus has been more on diversity and culture and not the health disparities seen in different cultures and minoritised groups (Bass-Haugen 2009), nor institutional racism in the profession, suggesting that occupational therapists contribute to the continuation of the racial inequalities and health inequities.

There is limited literature in occupational therapy focusing on health disparities between communities, and in 1988 already Cassidy urged colleagues within the profession to increase research on health disparities and examine how current health systems were perpetuating health disparities (Cassidy 1988). Over the last few decades, dialogue in occupational therapy and occupational science has evolved to a broader understanding of socio-cultural and socio-political influences on occupational performance (Iwama 2006; Watson 2006; Pollard *et al.* 2009); moreover, epistemology to guide in addressing the issues is still limited. In addition, in the national healthcare system in many countries around the world, occupational therapists are still required to focus more on the individual's health rather than the health of a population or family. However, this is not the case in Brazil, where they practise social occupational therapy, a political and ethical framework for practice that works not only with individuals, but also alongside communities, and with systems to enable human, social and occupational rights for those experiencing conditions that are socially disadvantaging them from thriving (Barros *et al.* 2005; Lopes & Malfitano 2020).

The second consideration to discuss is that Nelson (2007), reflecting on work by Dickie (2004), said that occupational therapy's worldview is western and only becomes aware of cultures outside this when faced with the 'other' that is not of the western culture. Occupational therapists from dominant cultures, such as the Global North, can be considered culturally blind if they deem their own values and beliefs to be the norm against which they analyse and compare during assessment and treatment (Whiteford & Wilcock 2000). The same could be attributed to racism in occupational therapy; the clinician's worldview aligning with the dominant Eurocentric and North American populations and culture could govern/influence their interpretation of problems and dysfunctions experienced by persons and groups from different heritage and cultural backgrounds, for example BIPOC groups.

The third aspect to consider is why occupational therapists would work in inequitable health systems without appearing to say anything about it. The answer is multifactorial. It could be related to various issues, including disempowerment of occupational therapists in traditionally hierarchical health and social care systems; the strength of identity of the profession dominated by the medical model; the professional bodies globally not making it part of their strategic agendas, and being involved in politics which is part of being involved in social justice. Occupational therapy is the invisible or lesser-known profession compared to medical doctors, nursing and physiotherapy, therefore it just tries to fit in with the dominating professions (Turner & Knight 2015; Walder et al. 2022). Some current curricula do not adequately include teaching social justice and equity and the students/practitioners therefore lack the theoretical and actionable knowledge and attention on social and cultural issues and public health they need to address racism and collaboratively create change. The occupational therapy students complete practice placements in services that are inequitable and unjust without questioning, thus they maintain the status quo of structural racism and discrimination when they become qualified occupational therapists. Occupational therapy is a white-dominated profession which has maintained the status quo because it is easier to carry on as it is and continuously recycle the same white and colonial ideology and systems.

Lastly, in 2000, Ramugondo reasoned that the under-representation of occupational therapists from minoritised or oppressed communities might be why we, as a profession, have not engaged in topics like racism and inequities. Ramugondo (2000) highlighted that knowledge created depends on who created the knowledge. If we do not have a diverse professional population from different parts of the world and heritage backgrounds who have experienced racism, marginalization and health inequity, as a profession we will not be motivated to advocate for and make changes, other than piecemeal transient actions for pockets of individuals or groups trying to work on this without the full backing of the professional bodies and profession. This is hard work – doing the right thing is hard work, and the easy stance is to do nothing, to stay as we are.

Role of occupational therapy to reduce the impact of health disparities due to systemic racism

Discussions on health disparities and social determinants are in the public health domain, hence there needs to be more content in occupational therapy curricula that addresses these issues (Dougall & Buck 2021). Clinical training placements should include the topics as part of assessments, which will keep the topics 'alive' in practice. Occupational therapy training courses should include influencing public health policies through national professional bodies and challenging systems that perpetuate health disparities. Lavalley and Robinson Johnson (2022) suggest that collective action by the occupational fraternity is needed. Moreover, evidence through research must be provided on the impact of attending to or not attending to social determinants of health, on health equity, and the influence it has on people's ability to perform needed occupations, such as work and schooling.

Occupational justice is part of social justice, which is in the realms of politics. Occupational therapy professional bodies need to encourage, support and guide their members on how to become more politically aware and how to actively influence politicians locally, regionally and nationally. Strategies to increase health equity include advocacy and creating opportunity for minoritised and marginalised service user groups to empower themselves so that they can also advocate for themselves. Again, in curricula, students should be exposed to topics such as racism in health and social care, the politics of health and social care, campaigning, being activists, as well as the usual topic of advocacy; the term advocacy seems relatable to saviourism.

In occupational therapy, we need to critically review our underlying assumptions, theories, models and frameworks to ensure that they are relevant tools to use with all populations and that we progress from the traditions of western-worldview values and whiteness to imbuing the social justice and human rights attributes the profession professes to be built on. As guidance, we should look at following the advice of Williams and de Witt (2020), who said that in rehabilitation we should address the social determinants of health and social inequities that people are facing in navigating their everyday lives. Identifying and creating theories, models, tools and frameworks reflective of diverse cultures and values should be a priority of the profession so that clinicians are equipped to provide health interventions for a diverse population. Curricula sessions or modules could be co-designed with members from minoritised or marginalised groups, thus ensuring their voices are centred and heard within the teaching and learning process.

It is important to increase the diversity of heritage backgrounds among the occupational therapy population to be reflective of the public population seen. A diverse body of occupational therapists might take more cognizance of inequalities and inequities; however, skills training on these topics should be part of the occupational therapy education and for clinicians post qualification. Understanding occupational injustice risk factors, the transactional nature of occupational engagement and the influence of socio-political, socio-economical and socio-cultural aspects on occupational engagement is essential for all occupational therapists to enable their practice to deliver equity. A focus by national occupational therapist associations on issues of justice and the political nature of engagement in healthy occupations of choice, and awareness around occupational justice, equity issues and the impact it has on healthcare provision, are needed. Getting involved and having a say in health management and governance at institutional, local and country level should be business as usual for occupational therapists.

Racism and health inequities lead to chronic stress and other chronic co-morbidities, which creates additional costs for health, social care and justice systems, among others. We need a trauma-informed approach in our practice and curricula. This is because living with racism, discrimination, inequity and injustice harms humans, and as occupational therapists we need to understand this and engage with it if we are going to be effective for humanity.

Conclusion

There needs to be a review of health, welfare and social policy to truly address the social determinants of health and promote justice and equity using the lens of antiracist practice. We need to draw on existing Global South and indigenous understandings of health and wellbeing, and centre the voices of the minoritised and marginalised – the very people harmed by racism and oppressed by the continuing colonialist ideology – to enhance the health and social care system, to innovate our profession and the services we deliver and to disrupt the status quo of institutional racist reproduction. Occupational therapists are well placed to lead and contribute to such policies, as we are dual trained in physical and mental health and work in a huge variety of settings and services. We have skills in transformation because that is what our guiding philosophy, knowledge and training enable us to apply in our work in collaboration with people and communities. We need to get vocal, active and political about injustices, rather than contributing to the continuation of the status quo of racial inequalities and health inequities. There is no time to waste, and it is urgent that we as a profession get involved effectively right now, not later.

Reflective quadrant: Identifying, recording and understanding learning from the chapter

What? (Describe what have I learnt)	**Relevance?** (Why is this topic relevant to me/to my practice? Relate/align to/with, e.g., research literature, professional bodies' proficiencies/competencies, service delivery/service user benefit, legislation – briefly and critically discuss)
How will this learning change me/my practice?	**What actions do I have to follow up on to develop my learning in this area or apply to my practice?** (SMART goal format or similar)

— CHAPTER 4 —

Antiracist Occupational Therapy Education: Perspectives from Ghana, the United Kingdom, and the United States of America

Khalilah Robinson Johnson, Selena Washington,
Eric Nkansah Opoku, Ellen Serwaa Adomako

This chapter provides international perspectives from occupational therapy educators in the United States of America (United States), the United Kingdom (UK) and Ghana on the impact of colonisation in the development of an imperialist western occupational therapy education; the call for antiracist occupational therapy curricula globally; and strategies for implementing antiracist concepts and methods in occupational therapy academic programmes. The late Desmond Tutu's sage words remind us of the importance of education for a just society:

> Inclusive, good-quality education is a foundation for dynamic and equitable societies. (Tutu & Van Roekel 2010)

Critical questions guiding this chapter are:

- What is the impact of colonisation on occupational therapy education?

- How are antiracist concepts and strategies embedded in current occupational therapy theoretical frameworks?

- How can occupational therapy academic programmes demonstrate a commitment to antiracism and tackle race inequality through critical pedagogical approaches?

Introduction

The World Federation of Occupational Therapists (WFOT) established minimum standards for occupational therapy programmes in 1958, with its most recent revision to these standards occurring in 2016 (WFOT 2016). The WFOT (2016) affirmed the intent of the standards was to '... advance human rights in global society by impacting the profession through the establishment of international standards...' (p.3) and '[to expand] the perspective of the education of occupational therapists to prepare them for a global professional community' (p.10). It was agreed on by the occupational therapy international community to commit to standards that centred social, educational and professional concerns. Although the WFOT minimum standards are not required for academic programmes, many of the standards are subsumed in the missions and educational philosophies of individual programmes around the world. The nations and educational systems the authors of this chapter represent are loosely aligned to the social consciousness-raising standards set forth by the WFOT, which, arguably, may have a direct impact on if and how occupational therapy programmes address culture, coloniality and structural factors that impact occupation.

Although the authors represent occupational therapy academic programmes in different global geographical, cultural and socio-political contexts, their programmes share a commitment to transformative educational practices rooted in cultural humility and culturally affirming pedagogies[1] aimed to prepare students to enter into the diversity of practices available in occupational therapy. It is imperative that occupational therapy programmes prepare students to enter practice that reflects the concerns and needs of a global society. This commitment is a prerequisite to instituting pedagogical practices that address imperialism and racism in occupational therapy education (Sakellariou & Pollard 2013).

Racism and occupational therapy curriculum

Coloniality refers to the destruction of indigenous and cultural traditions, education and knowledge systems, and other social forms and ways of being as a result of colonialisation (Laing 2021; Wane & Todd

---

1   Pedagogy – theory and method of teaching and learning.

2018). Education was central to colonialisation (Wane & Todd 2018), as notions where racially minoritised 'others' (e.g. indigenous and enslaved peoples) were viewed as inferior and were normalised. These normalisations are the results of deep-seated racist logic and systems of knowing (Lavalley & Robinson Johnson 2022). Colonial epistemology privileges scholars of the North and West, mostly racialised as white, and the knowledge they produce in the 'theoretical apparatus' by inferiorising the rest (Grosfoguel 2011; Hammell 2011; Kronenberg 2020b). This includes privileging languages, particularly English, and conceptualisations and narratives of occupation as well as standards for teaching and practising occupational therapy (Pollard & Sakellariou 2012; Sakellariou & Pollard 2012).

Hence, decolonising, as defined by Pirbhai-Illich *et al.* (2017), is the process of exposing the structures and systemic traumas that create inequities among indigenous and other diverse groups, including the erasure of their knowledge systems. It includes disrupting the dominance of western centric ideologies and making visible the knowledges that have been invisible and excluded for equity and justice (Pirbhai-Illich *et al.* 2017). The goal of decolonial education movements is to refocus attention to other knowledges by taking up various emancipatory struggles, which includes, but is not limited to, historical and contemporary socio-political movements of indigenous and Black people (Laing 2021). Although it is beyond the scope of this chapter, it is important to note that decolonisation does not occur at the level of pedagogy exclusively; rather, decolonising requires responses at multiple sites (e.g. curricular, research, institutional and policy levels) within and outside the educational enterprise (Bhambra *et al.* 2018; Pirbhai-Illich *et al.* 2017) and a constant critical examination of the Eurocentric discourses and ideologies that pervade our knowledge systems.

It is imperative that occupational therapy lecturers acknowledge and engage their and other racialised systems of knowing and experiences of the world as their identities, cultural heritage and positionalities among others are inextricably linked to the processes and outcomes of educational instruction. Therefore, to circumvent further perpetuation of privileging the dominant culture's voices and ideologies and universal truths about knowing and doing occupation, intentions must be given to recognising and disrupting hegemonic practices (speaking specifically to education in the context of this text) (Pirbhai-Illich *et al.* 2017; Ramugondo 2018). This includes emphasising the power of different knowledges (ways of knowing) and pedagogical orientations by enlivening knowledges that fall outside the colonial complex (Ramugondo 2018); and reclaiming and validating indigenous and other ways of knowing (Laing 2021).

In the context of occupational therapy education, by incorporating antiracist pedagogical methods and strategies, educators are transparent about the historical role that western epistemology and educational practices have played and continue to play in the development of occupational therapy around the world, not only in perpetuating racism and discrimination against many minoritized cultural groups, but also in denying heterogeneity in knowing and engaging occupations. This articulates to the broader issues of cultural imperialism, systemic and institutional racism, colonialism, privileging colonial thinking, and requires a critical and reflexive examination of systems at all levels, ourselves as occupational therapy educators and practitioners, and our efforts towards transformational change.

Developing and instituting an antiracist occupational therapy curriculum

Occupational therapy practice and education developed and spread to other global geographical areas since its inception in the United States. People have trained in the profession through learning exchanges abroad and/or with renowned occupational therapy educators offering the training to host institutions. Dr Elizabeth Casson is referenced as starting the formal training of occupational therapists in England after a study visit to the United States in 1925, followed by Alice Constance Tebbit (and later Glyn Owens) from the UK completing an occupational therapy programme of study at the Philadelphia School of Occupational Therapy. India (All India Occupational Therapists' Association (AIOTA) 2018) and Ghana (Ndaa 2014) have reported similar patterns of people training in the United States and UK respectively before establishing occupational therapy programmes in their country. In South Africa, two pioneering occupational therapy practitioners from Britain helped to advance the occupational therapy programme (Occupational Therapy Association of South Africa 2018). Issues to consider with this approach include the relevance and the applicability of such knowledge to the practitioner's own country's context on return, as most global occupational therapy courses are based on Eurocentric knowledge. Owens (1960, cited by Tyldesley 2004) acknowledged that there could be 'no direct transfer' of the knowledge acquired from studying in the United States to the training programme in the UK due to the differences in the 'educational, social, cultural and economic pattern' (Owens 1960: 14 as cited by Tyldesley 2004).

Occupational science and occupational therapy scholars, as well as post-colonial and post-modern thinkers, have noted that knowledge and how we engage and enact that knowledge is influenced by our belief systems and positionalities (Alcoff 1991; Hammell 2011; Kupperman 2001; Said 1993). It is understood that curricula designs in non-western countries are informed by experts from western countries (Melese & Tadege 2019; Agho & John 2017; Krefting 1992); therefore, it is critical to be conscious of the fact that westernised ideas, theories, models and assumptions may inevitably crowd the content of these curricula if critical reflexivity is not exercised. Perhaps, this could be one of the means through which westernised occupational therapy is being propagated and theoretical imperialism, intellectual colonialism and racism perpetuated (Grenier 2020; Simaan 2020a; Whalley Hammell 2019; Ramugondo 2015; Whalley Hammell & Iwama 2012; Hammell 2011; Hammell 2009; Ife 2008).

This is of enormous importance because just as an apple tree bears apples, so shall a westernised curriculum bear 'westernised' occupational therapy practitioners. Consequently, occupational therapy assessments and interventions informed by contextually irrelevant theories, models and assumptions are likely to be inappropriate, inadequate and oppressive (Al Busaidy & Borthwick 2012; Whalley Hammell 2019; Iwama 2003, 2005; Uys & Samuels 2010). For occupational therapy practitioners to give full expression to the great idea of the profession and for service consumers to benefit from the uniqueness of the profession everywhere in the world, it is important that the content of the educational curricula and professional training is culturally relevant.

Antiracist concepts, methods and pedagogy

Krishnagiri and colleagues (2017) discussed within their qualitative analysis that what and how you are taught regarding occupation is what you will practise. The central argument is that occupational science and occupational therapy curricula must be contextualised, culturally relevant, responsive and inclusive of global perspectives. As Creek (2010) summarised, academic programmes must utilise the specific language, concepts and theoretical guideposts and frameworks to dismantle colonialism and western practices within occupational science and occupational therapy. Occupational therapy academic programmes based on an English language curricula and western societal norms and values are one of the main challenges non-western academic institutions face in the cultural translation and application of fundamental occupational therapy concepts within diverse populations (Creek 2010; Malkawi *et al.* 2020). Western cultural norms and ideologies have formulated the core concepts of the profession, creating dominant cultural perspectives, models and theoretical guideposts which mirror the values of the western perspectives (Malkawi *et al.* 2020; Whalley Hammell 2019).

Antiracist occupational therapy curricula will be grounded and generated through the learning of marginalised populations utilising a critical reflexive educational practice (Kinsella & Whiteford 2009), which moves beyond individual experiences and encompasses the power dynamic of race and (white) privilege within society (Simaan 2020b). There is a need to increase students' critical consciousness of the diverse occupational needs of marginalised populations, and students' understanding of occupational therapy practice and justice concepts (Aldrich & Peters 2019; Kronenberg 2020b; Ramugondo 2015; Simaan 2020a); yet, there is a dearth of antiracist occupation-centred educational methodology and conceptual published material from the Global North (United States, Canada and Europe, Israel, Asia, Australia and New Zealand) and Global South (Africa, Latin America and the Caribbean, Pacific Islands, developing parts of Asia and the Middle East) (Grenier *et al.* 2020; Mahoney & Kiraly-Alvarez 2019; Simaan 2020b).

The inclusion of non-western global perspectives, occupation-centred methodology and theoretical concepts is vital to deconstruct and understand antiracist ways of doing, being, becoming and belonging within society (Wilcock 2006). However, the relationship between occupation and cultural aspects of 'doing, being, becoming and belonging' which compass the intersectionality of social class, race, gender, sexual orientation, religion and disability, has only been partially explored within academic spaces (Grenier *et al.* 2020; Laliberte-Rudman *et al.*

2008; Sakellariou & Pollard 2013; Wilcock 2006). Further, antiracist methodologies exemplify the potential for educators and researchers to challenge coloniality and support diverse perspectives within occupational science and occupational therapy curricula and practice (Huff *et al.* 2020).

Cultural humility, along with critical reflexivity, provides a mechanism through which to systematically recognize the cultural differences that are present among diverse clients and populations who do not identify with dominant western cultural groups (Beagan 2020; Hammell 2013; Kinsella & Whiteford 2009; Muñoz 2007). Exposure to and recognition of the intersects between cultural influences and identities challenges students to engage in self-reflection and the acknowledgement of occupational therapy's role in addressing social inequities and power imbalances that exist within society (Beagan 2018; Mahoney & Kiraly-Alvarez 2019).

Examples of occupational science and occupational therapy frameworks to facilitate antiracist occupational therapy

Occupational consciousness

Ramugondo (2015), through the construct of occupational consciousness, specifically analyses the conscious and unconscious state of the profession which embraces and promotes independence and western ideology, with limited regard of those who lack access to societal resources (i.e. healthcare, living wage, housing and education). Within the classroom setting, students are able to utilise this construct to identify and deconstruct the power dynamics between therapists and clients and communities who engage with occupational therapy; along with the lecturer's ability to challenge dominant practices taught as a part of western ideology. The utilisation of this construct can assist in transformative processes of what is taught in academic programmes, where and why research is conducted, and how students enter the profession as reflexive and empathetic practitioners.

Cultural responsiveness

Cultural responsiveness and culturally responsive care in occupational therapy refers to a contextualised and equitable approach that centres the shared experiences and meaningful occupations of diverse populations (Muñoz 2007). Cultural responsiveness involves a critical reflection and awareness of the differences in power and privilege and the inequalities that exist within society, which places cultural knowledge on the same level as the development of skills and behaviours when designing curricula (Muñoz 2007; Talero et al. 2015). Talero and colleagues (2015) introduced the Culturally Responsive Care in Occupational Therapy embedded in Service-Learning (CRCOT-SL) model. This educational model integrates three concepts within entry-level occupational therapy education: 1) occupational perspective of population health (Wilcock 2006); 2) a conceptualisation of culturally relevant occupational therapy (Trentham et al. 2007); and 3) the Participatory Occupational Justice Framework (POJF) (Whiteford & Townsend 2010). CRCOT-SL follows a revised Bloom's taxonomy (Anderson & Krathwohl 2001), including learning the basic-to-complex application of responsiveness and a responsive healthcare approach, and addressing the occupational needs of individuals and communities within a local and/or global context. The application of the CRCOT through a service delivery model allows for advocacy of occupational opportunities in contexts which may be unfamiliar to students without perpetuating a history of colonisation and oppression (Simaan 2020a; Talero et al. 2015).

Ubuntu

Ubuntu is a South African philosophy which emphasises the collective occupational wellbeing of individuals and communities as a foundation to and focus of practice, where occupational needs are interactive, and interconnectedness of individuals and communities are in a 'constant shared process of becoming' (Cornell & Van Marle 2005; van Vuuren et al. 2020; Ramugondo & Kronenberg 2015: 12). The emphasis on the shared process of 'becoming' dismantles the individualistic ideology of independence which is central within the practice of occupational therapy in westernised practice (Ramugondo & Kronenberg 2015).

Occupational justice

Occupational justice, derived from social justice in response to a renewed commitment by the occupational therapy profession to address occupational needs, is a key component of examining conscious and unconscious biases as well as highlighting and reconstructing knowledge/

practice within occupational science and occupational therapy pedagogy (Durocher *et al.* 2014; Hess-April *et al.* 2016; Townsend & Wilcock 2004b). Occupational justice is achieved when occupational rights are enacted, and individuals/communities/populations are empowered to choose and perform occupations according to their own needs or wants (Townsend & Wilcock 2004b). Occupational therapy students are able to analyse and address the conceptualisations of occupational injustice, such as occupational apartheid, occupational alienation, occupational marginalisation and occupational imbalance, along with systemic power issues within practice contexts (Durocher *et al.* 2014; Townsend & Wilcock 2004b; Townsend & Whiteford 2005). Within the classroom, lecturers can attend to critical perspectives and raise ethical, moral, civic, financial and philosophical questions about injustice and the tensions or gaps between ideals and reality (ought vs. is) of individuals/communities living with inequitable disadvantages of oppression (Hess-April *et al.* 2016; Mahoney & Kiraly-Alvarez 2019).

An example of developing an antiracist curriculum

The document, *Introduction to Antiracist Curriculum Development,* by the Coalition for Racial Equality and Rights (2021) outlined practical steps with resources to support educators in providing an antiracist curriculum. Although it was developed for schools in Scotland, the principles discussed are applicable in occupational therapy education. Laing (2021: 6), from a critical pedagogical approach, argued that it is 'not only *what* we teach, but *how*' we teach it that helps ensure an antiracist approach has been adopted.

1. *Ensure a diversity of teaching staff, not just reading lists.* In instances where there is no diversity of the teaching staff, the institution should make a conscious effort with budget allocation to invite guest lecturers. Laing (2021) iterated that this should not be just any scholar but those with alternative epistemology that could help foster the agenda of an antiracist approach to curriculum. The downside of this suggestion could be the cost implication; but alternative approaches, like the use of online teaching and learning platforms, can be considered while acknowledging the benefit of face-to-face instruction.

2. *Enable antiracist pedagogies by having a horizontal relationship between student and educator* (e.g. student-led workshop).

3. *Encourage social justice, liberation and antiracism* by teaching to encourage students to develop antiracist praxis.

4. *Antiracist student assessment criteria.* As much as possible, assessment methods should be varied such that the strengths of various students in the programmes can be highlighted. A combination of examination, written assignments, oral presentations and practical assessment is recommended not just across curriculum but for modules. The assessments should be supported using an antiracist marking criteria rubric (Inoue 2015). Overall, the 'marking criteria for the module should reflect the students' commitment to using reading that acknowledged contributions from a greater range of thinkers' (Laing 2021: 13).

5. *Centre antiracism in the development and delivery of the curriculum* and not simply as an add-on. Antiracist pedagogy is both a framework and a process.

(Coalition for Racial Equality and Rights 2021)

AUTHOR'S VOICE: ELLEN – offering a child with cerebral palsy a shower

This recount of my experience shows how institutional racism in occupational therapy course structure and content impacted my learning and my feelings of belonging to occupational therapy in the UK context.

Between 2008 and 2010, I was an international student from Ghana in the UK pursuing a master's degree in occupational therapy (pre-registration). My mission was simple – to complete the required coursework, qualify as an occupational therapist, gain some work experience and return to my home country to help establish an occupational therapy programme. This journey, however, began like most international students simultaneously navigating the new cultural context and the demands of rigorous coursework, including visa issues, stipend delays and placement challenges.

Focusing on the teaching and learning, I was fortunate to find myself in a small cohort of six other students, of whom three were international students. I immediately became aware of the differences in the teaching style of my university compared to how I was trained in Ghana when I pursued a Bachelor of Arts in Psychology. I devised strategies to adapt and to be able to catch up with coursework. However, in hindsight, what I actually experienced was a difficulty to fully comprehend what was being delivered. No, I did not have a learning disability if you were to ask; rather, the issue was what I would refer to as the 'jargon' that was used in the delivery of the sessions. By this, I do not mean the complex medical terminologies but the words people in England use daily. For example, having a bath versus having a shower, and understanding the structure of the National Health Service (NHS). In the context of activity analysis, understanding the difference between 'to have a shower' and 'to have a bath' was necessary as there were different steps and equipment involved to complete these activities. What I was familiar with was to have a shower or get a bucket with water to complete my washing. Therefore, I responded that I would offer the child with cerebral palsy a shower.

It was the same when lecturers began to talk in class about the various healthcare settings like residential and nursing home care and sometimes other basic things like a client home environment. I was in student accommodation and not privy to the design of most homes in the UK. The lecturer's application of occupational consciousness (Ramugondo 2015) or the CRCOT-SL (Talero et al. 2015) approach to teaching, I think, would have helped me overcome most of the challenges faced. To the lecturer, what I am recounting could be common knowledge or something that students from the UK readily know. However, I felt there could have been further discussions around the activity of washing oneself and the different ways this can be done; then, intentionally invite different perspectives where I could share my experience. An acknowledgement of my approach to washing would have helped me to fully understand that the occupational therapy theories that I was learning in the UK would be applicable to the Ghana context.

I chose to share this 'somewhat simple' everyday knowledge within England that I struggled with and that impacted on my learning. I had similar experiences when reading textbooks – sometimes I struggled to fully comprehend the context of what was written. Conversely, this could be the experience of a student from another country who finds themselves in Ghana. What I am suggesting is that lecturers/tutors should acknowledge how their curriculum has been designed, consider the diversity of students, and invite different perspectives. This would boost student confidence and their understanding of what is being taught. For me, I recognised some of these difficulties in time, and worked with a tutor who advocated for additional support. In hindsight, there should have been more support available within the university for international students; if this was available, I was not aware of it.

AUTHOR'S VOICE: SELENA – facilitating classroom assignments and discussions through occupational science/therapy research and practice

The written class assignment, focusing on critical perspectives of 'isms' through occupational science/occupational therapy (OS/OT) literature, utilises the characteristics of social identity (Harro 2000) and the cycle of socialisation. The 'ism', by definition denotes a basis for prejudice or discrimination and how this may intersect with other unjust societal 'isms' such as race-ism, class-ism, sex-ism and age-ism. This assignment is designed to extend students' knowledge of humans as diverse occupational beings through an intersection of social identities (i.e. race, class, gender, religion, disability and sexuality), and can illuminate antiracist practices. The OS/OT literature provided to the students encourages them to explore topics of oppressions and marginalisation based on a person's social identity and the intersections of identity.

Through the lens of antiracist practice, culture, occupation and justice, students are able to engage with the literature, critically analyse dominant societal practices and perspectives, and articulate arguments regarding the need for cultural responsibility, sensitivity and humility when forming therapeutic relationships with others. Along with this is the utilisation of active learning strategies where students engage with content related to occupational justice and occupational science constructs, for example *consciousness and possibilities* toward current and/ or long-standing societal, cultural and racial issues (Galvaan *et al.* 2015; Ramugondo 2015). Examples of the literature used for different topics within the assignment include racism (Beagan 2020; Lavalley & Robinson Johnson 2022), sexism (Kingsley & Molineux 2000), transphobia

(Dowers *et al.* 2019), ableism (Yañez & Zúñiga 2018), classism (Beagan *et al.* 2018) and ageism (Friedman & VanPuymbrouck 2021). The objectives of the assignment are as follows (but could be developed to focus primarily on racism):

1. Critically reflect on the 'ism' that is being examined/analysed/discussed within the article, what social identity or intersection/s of identity is directly targeted; and does this or how can this intersect with antiracist practice.

2. Describe the author's point of view of the 'ism' that has been taught and or enforced in society, which influences bias and/or prejudice (or could add 'discrimination'), and directly or indirectly influences engagement in meaningful occupation.

3. How does the author(s) support or expound on the 'ism' through the use of other scholars' work?

4. Discuss what areas of the article resonated with you most (and why) and describe the links you see between an occupational perspective (i.e. occupational constructs and/or occupational justice) and 'isms'.

AUTHOR'S VOICE: ERIC – 'I prefer the white occupational therapist, not you'

In 2020, I took part in virtual discussions with Dr Frank Kronenberg on racism and its impact on human occupation, health and wellbeing, including his eminent Occupational Therapy Association of Ghana Congress 2020 keynote, 'Undoing colonial-OT (Coloniality): Occupational therapy cultivating a praxis of doing well together in Ghana (Kronenberg 2020a)'. I experienced a critical awakening to how racism continues to be perpetuated on African soils.

For example, I reflected on Sefa (a pseudonym), one of the participants of my master's research project, which explored the transition from student to health professional by the first cohort of locally trained occupational therapists in Ghana (Opoku *et al.* 2022). In one discussion, Sefa recounted an experience which she described as 'traumatizing'.

Sefa was a Ghanaian female occupational therapist who, as a new graduate, was excited about putting her knowledge, skills and experience into practice in paediatrics. Sefa described that the majority of the children were white, and their parents were actively involved in all therapy sessions. She was the only Black practitioner on the occupational therapy team. Sefa recounted an event which made her lose interest in working in the school. A new student, a child with Down syndrome whose parents were British expatriates, was admitted, and as customary an initial assessment was required, which was assigned to Sefa. Sefa recounted on initially meeting the child and parents, 'They responded to my greetings, but the mother of the child asked me why the other occupational therapist was not attending to them (referring to a white occupational therapist) but rather me.' Sefa continued, 'I told them the therapist they preferred was busy with other children but the woman told me she had all the time to wait for the therapist she preferred. I did not understand why the woman was hostile to me even though it was her first time meeting me.' Sefa proposed to Cindy (pseudonym for the occupational therapist the new student's mother preferred) to switch clients with her, but Cindy did not know the parent. Sefa did complain to her management but heard nothing back and was sure nothing was done about it. As the environment was not conducive for her to flourish, she later left the school.

Reflecting on Sefa's words, it is clear that she experienced interpersonal racism. I am reading more about this and taking part in and facilitating discussions on antiracism in occupational therapy. Racism has always existed in Ghana but has not been integrated into occupational therapy education discussions. Integrating discussion on racism into the curriculum will help students develop an awareness of racism in practice as well as strategies to initiate concrete antiracist actions (Sterman & Njelesani 2021).

Conclusion

Antiracist occupation-centred education and conceptual frameworks create a bridge to cultural knowledge and lived experiences globally, enhancing the curriculum. To be able to engage in an antiracist occupational therapy curriculum, first you must understand what the meaning of this is, why you want to use it, what the key principles are and how you can approach the transformation of the curriculum using this method.

You must engage with what you will be centring and decentring, and how and why, and really interrogate your decisions and actions, at the same time keeping a check on whether you are still following antiracism principles. Antiracist methodologies exemplify the potential to challenge coloniality, disrupt racism and support the enhancement of occupational therapy curricula and practice by integrating Black, Global South and indigenous knowledges, collaborating with professionals, researchers, service users and students in delivering these curricula (Huff *et al.* 2020). Antiracism is action to transform curricula, to cultivate an environment where staff, students and institutions can work from a global perspective, collaborating and integrating Black, Global South and indigenous people and communities and their knowledges, so that those very colonial power structures and hierarchies that disadvantage and discriminate are seen and hence disrupted for the benefit of all in education. It is through this lens that lecturers can cultivate diverse populations in academic programmes and classrooms where students can develop antiracist responsiveness in their therapeutic approach and professional practice.

Reflective quadrant: Identifying, recording and understanding learning from the chapter

What? (Describe what have I learnt)

Relevance? (Why is this topic relevant to me/to my practice? Relate/align to/with, e.g., research literature, professional bodies' proficiencies/competencies, service delivery/service user benefit, legislation – briefly and critically discuss)

How will this learning change me/my practice?

What actions do I have to follow up on to develop my learning in this area or apply to my practice? (SMART goal format or similar)

CHAPTER 5

Experiences of Racism in Occupational Therapy Clinical Placement Settings

Sherrille Tayson, Oliver Miller, Valentine Tendai
Mutsvairo, Musharrat J. Ahmed-Landeryou

Introduction

For occupational therapy students, it is fundamental to undertake clinical training placements. This is where the students apply their learned knowledge from the taught elements of the course, and practise applying it to real-life, thus gaining exposure to the realities and complexities of contemporary health and social care provision. Clinical placements prepare the students for entry into the profession as a qualified practitioner. How the students experience and are impacted by the people helping with their training is important, and has consequences, as Professor Maya Angelou tells us that from her experience to take heed,

> I've learned that people will forget what you said, people will forget what you did, but people will never forget how you made them feel.[1]

Clinical training from placement begins to develop the student's professional identity (Turner & Knight 2015), professional socialisation abilities (Kerin 2020), personal management qualities and lifelong learning skills to thrive once qualified (Parker & Badger 2018). The process of being an occupational therapy student is both challenging and fulfilling. To qualify as an occupational therapist there are several processes that a student is required to overcome to demonstrate their theoretical understanding

---

[1] Quote posted on her Twitter account, 2018, https://twitter.com/DrMayaAngelou/status/1036327789488734208

and clinical competencies (Golos & Tekuzener 2019). Throughout the degree process, a student's knowledge and understanding will be assessed in a variety of ways. These may include essays, written exams, presentations and performance on clinical training placements. This chapter focuses on some of the lived experiences of the authors, who identify as racialised as Black and are British, during their time on occupational therapy placements as students. The authors graduated between one and four years ago.

The critical questions that guide this chapter are:

- How does racism manifest in occupational therapy placements?

- How can occupational therapy courses ensure equity of placement experience?

Background

Throughout the years of studying occupational therapy, students are required to have practice placements in a variety of settings (WFOT 2016). Practice placements for students can be very stressful for a variety of reasons (Spiliotopoulou 2007). However, for occupational therapy students from Black, Asian or minoritised ethnicities (BAME) heritages there are often additional stresses, which we will explore further in the chapter. According to Bonilla-Silva (2014: 302), the healthcare setting has become a symbolic expression of 'white dominance'. Although Bonilla-Silva (2014) focuses on racial inequality in the United States, we can presume that as occupational therapists work in healthcare and some of what Bonilla-Silva is identifying is in healthcare, then this could be true experientially for BAME practitioner groups in occupational therapy. Data from the UK Workforce Race and Equality Standards (WRES) shows similar institutional racism – white dominance – and outcomes for BAME populations in NHS employee careers (NHS England 2021). Occupational therapists are required to work within the specific policies and legal frameworks that govern their professional practice. However, according to Smedley (2012), these policies and legal frameworks are often the result of discrimination, racial bias and stereotyping because they are based on white supremacy ideology. If this is going on for qualified occupational therapy professionals, then what's not to say that some occupational therapy students from BAME groups must be experiencing the outcomes from institutional racism while on practice placements?

AUTHOR'S VOICE: SHERRILLE'S PLACEMENT EXPERIENCE – microaggression

Placement was the part of the course that I used to look forward to as it's an opportunity to apply practically the theoretical knowledge taught at university. I'm a creative and practical person, so placement was my favourite part of the course. I had already been on a previous placement in a community occupational therapy setting, which I thoroughly enjoyed. But unfortunately, this wasn't the case on my second placement, which was on an acute mental health ward. Before I inform you of my placement experience, I want to add that at the time I was pregnant, and I have an invisible chronic condition which affects my whole body, especially when I'm in stressful situations. The university placement team was aware of these facts.

The placement started oddly, when I first arrived and met my practice educator and abruptly she told me that she couldn't believe I was her student, despite me showing proof. She was the opposite of welcoming and proceeded to instruct me to wait in the canteen for over an hour while she confirmed the placement with the university. I was confused because we had been emailing one another prior to the start of placement. I felt something was off; she made me feel like a burden throughout the duration of my placement, with frequent minor digs at my abilities and appearance. On many occasions, I was ignored whenever I greeted her; at times, she would give me a blank stare and turn away from me or just suddenly leave the office when I spoke to her. In addition to this, she wouldn't allow me to shadow her or accompany her on visits. However, she would happily volunteer to give that opportunity to another occupational therapy student, who was there with her own practice educator. It quickly became clear that I would have to direct and map my own learning experience.

During one supervision, I used this opportunity to discuss my concerns with my educator. I was ridiculed and told I was being jealous of the other occupational therapy student; all the concerns I raised were ignored. As placement progressed, my educator would put me in dangerous situations, for example on the ward, and countless times after that she would leave the office door ajar when exiting the office, when it was advised that doors to offices should be shut at all times. On my first day when my educator had left the office door ajar, and I hadn't noticed, I was shocked when a patient ran into the office and sat on my lap. I was taken aback and if I'm honest, I felt scared. I felt unsafe and fearful often on this placement, especially for my unborn baby. I felt the educator's uncaring behaviour was specifically targeted towards me. Another example was when she told me on two occasions to attend a training which was outside the hospital, and she emphasised repeatedly that I must get there 20 minutes before the training or I would be refused entry. So, knowing this, I made sure I gave myself enough time to get to the training; when I arrived, I was told by my educator that she hadn't registered me or that it was on another day. When I informed my educator of these mishaps she laughed at me and said, 'Oh well, at least you had the chance to have a bit of a walk.'

Moreover, not long after all that running around, I began spotting during the placement, and that weekend, I was rushed to hospital and unfortunately I had a miscarriage. Due to the severity of the situation, I was admitted to hospital and rushed to theatre. I was heartbroken. I had made many preparations for the arrival of my baby. I resumed placement as usual the following Monday, as I felt I needed to keep busy, and I couldn't cope being home alone with my thoughts and the baby's things. I felt so much anger towards my educator; imagine having to smile at the person you believe was potentially a contributing reason as to why I had lost my baby. I couldn't help but believe the unnecessary stress and the running around from my educator contributed to the loss of my pregnancy. I continued my placement, but it was not easy putting on a smile and then in my lunchbreaks, crying in private. One day, I received a call from the mortuary to discuss the burial arrangements during placement. I couldn't concentrate the whole day; it became too much for me and I burst into tears in the bathroom. One of the occupational therapy assistants, a Black woman, found me crying and comforted me and informed me that my educator was not an easy person to work with.

I was thankful when my last week of placement was approaching, but unfortunately my educator was still treating me terribly. For example, she and I were assessing a patient in one of the rooms. This patient was very fond of me and looked to me for support as she answered the questions. As I was encouraging the patient to speak, my educator shushed me with her hand, her palm facing right in my face, and told me to be quiet. This was too much for me, as it was outright rude and very offensive in my culture for someone to put their left hand in my face. I decided that I needed intervention from a third party as soon as possible. So, I reported this incident to my educator's supervisor, who was approachable. I didn't report it to the university at that time, as I knew a few of my other friends who had challenges on placement had been withdrawn from their placements. I couldn't allow that as I had worked too hard. I explained everything to my educator's senior and expressed my worry that my educator might suddenly fail me out of spite. The educator's supervisor arranged for all three of us to sit down and for my educator to state in front of her that there was no possibility of her failing me at the end of the week. This gave me reassurance. Following on from my meeting with my educator and her supervisor, she used the last day of placement supervision to annihilate my character and interrogate me as to who told me to report her, and that she was sorry that I was not confident enough to speak to her. This was the last straw for me, and even though I passed placement, I decided to make a formal complaint.

All that had happened to me on placement was passed on to my course's placement team, and I thought I would get support from them, but it felt quite the opposite. I was told by a member of the practice placement team that I was potentially ruining the university's relationship with the placement and the chance for other students to go there, and what was the point of filing a formal complaint if I'd passed the practice placement. I was told that if I was to continue with this complaint, I would not have support from the university with this. I was shaken by the university placement team's reaction towards me, as in every placement briefing we were always reminded that the placement team had the students' best interests at heart. I did not experience this. It felt as if the placement team expected students, especially those from BAME populations, to work in unhealthy environments regardless, just to pass their placement. It's sad how many students from BAME groups are silenced because of the lack of support from their practice placement team.

After the placement, from my perspective, it seemed that some of the occupational therapy course staff were over-vigilant with me, scrutinizing my attendance, and so on. Even though the university staff were aware of what had happened to me with the miscarriage and practice placement, they continued to make my student life at university a perpetual stressful environment. At one point, I felt as if I wasn't supposed to be on the course any more, as I was told by a member of staff that my attendance was so low there was a risk of termination from the course. The truth of the case, from making my own enquiries with the absence team, confirmed that my attendance was exceptional, and once I passed this on to the course staff, they left this alone.

My reflective evaluation of the placement experience is that my practice educator was microaggressive daily because I am a Black woman. I didn't feel that the university placed any value on the trauma of the experience, and then further compounding my trauma by being hypervigilant with me. The literature suggests that my experience is the same as BAME populations in health and social care who report experiencing racism (King's Fund 2020; Gregory 2021).

AUTHOR'S VOICE: OLIVER'S PLACEMENT EXPERIENCE – fitting in

Throughout my process of qualifying to be an occupational therapist I was required to work in a range of different settings. These included community (physical), acute (physical), forensic (mental health) and paediatric settings. Each practice placement provided me with the ability to develop my skills and implement my theoretical knowledge. Pertaining to racial discrimination, there were certainly many occasions where I was made to feel uncomfortable due to being a Black man. These incidents were not specific to the practice educator, but would often be a result of communicating and interacting with the wider team. Throughout my life, I have experienced both individual and systemic racism due to the colour of my skin. Over the years this has come in many forms, including obvious verbal remarks about my heritage background, the colour of my skin, even down to the food I prefer to eat. More specifically, throughout my journey to become a qualified occupational therapist I have experienced a range of microaggressions that undoubtedly made the process of qualifying very difficult. According to Sue *et al.* (2007a, 2007b), racial microaggressions are the new face of racism and refer to accumulative humiliations, inappropriate jokes, attitudes and behaviours that individuals from BAME heritage face daily.

On every placement I completed I was always in the minority as a Black man. Moreover, on two of the four placements I was the only Black individual in the team. Naturally, this raised levels of anxiety based on what I have been through in the past as well as concerns relating to how the team and practice educator would take to me. Before you commence any placement your details are often sent to your practice educator in preparation. In many of my placements there were a variety of occasions where on first meeting my practice educator, or team members, they would express that I was not what they were 'expecting to see'. When challenged on this, some staff would say it was because I was a man; however, on some occasions staff had said to me it was because I am Black. Although to some this may not have been a problem, to me it often made me aware from the beginning of the placement that I was different. Moreover, I felt as though I needed to be increasingly conscious of how I engaged and communicated with the team to fit in. Although I did my best to be a part of the team, there were often many occasions where the team and I did not share common interests. This would immediately present barriers between me and the team and would impact the way in which I was treated. For example, I was told during a placement that I appeared to lack engagement and did not seem to make an effort to 'fit in'. When I discussed this further with my practice educator she used an example that at lunchtimes I would sometimes not sit with the team, opting to go for a walk. My practice educator went on to report that during the occasions where I did sit with the team at lunch, I would be reluctant to engage and appeared to be disinterested. I had to explain to my practice educator that unfortunately I did not watch the same TV programmes and did not share the same social interests as the others in the team, which impacted my ability to engage. Despite me explaining my reasons, it appeared I was being told that to pass the placement I would need to increase my level of engagement at lunchtimes with the team. This was not a practice placement learning outcome; I found this very difficult. I felt powerless, as when incidents like this occurred it often felt as though I was not being assessed on my skills competencies as an occupational therapy student.

As another example, during a specific placement I was required to complete an occupational therapy assessment with the support of my practice educator. This was the first assessment I was asked to lead during the placement, therefore I felt very anxious before starting. Within minutes of arriving at the property I was racially abused by the client. The client expressed that he did not like people like me and that I should go back to where I came from. My practice educator instantly took over the assessment, did not challenge the client and I was left to observe my educator from a distance. After the assessment, we didn't get to discuss the incident until three days later during supervision, whereupon I expressed how I was affected by what had happened. However, I was told by my educator (who is white) that this can happen with the older generation. She added that to fit in with occupational therapy I needed to have thick skin as this is something that would happen again in the future. This experience left me in a place of disbelief that my educator would not challenge the client's racist views and not be supportive towards me, thus invalidating my experience. At the time, I really felt that I should not continue in the profession, that I did not belong. I contemplated walking away. I felt unable to discuss the incident further with my practice educator as her communication showed she would not understand. However, I did discuss what happened and how I felt with a Black friend of mine who was in my cohort.

Reflecting on the placement experience from an antiracism lens, everyday racism experiences leave me with the sense of not belonging, which affected my feelings of safety and made me anxious, on edge. Belonging is a precursor for successful experience at university, and I struggled with fitting into the profession on placements, which is a reality for BAME population students (Hammond *et al.* 2019).

AUTHOR'S VOICE: VALENTINE'S PLACEMENT EXPERIENCE – stereotyping, oppressing, microaggressions

Since commencing the occupational therapy degree at university, I looked forward to committing my life to the profession I had chosen. After researching and hearing accounts of previous students studying occupational therapy, it appeared that practice placement was a highlight, an area to look forward to as part of the course. Set apart from the academic rigour of university assignments, I gathered placement was a haven to experience the reality of occupational therapy practice.

However, my experience on one of my practice placements didn't go too smoothly. I was assigned to a clinical educator, a charismatic, bubbly clinician who worked part-time, had ten years' clinical experience, and was eager to have a student under her wing. She mentioned that as soon as my name came up on the system, she was intrigued to be having an 'exotic person' briefly as part of the team. The prospect of a Black male occupational therapy student appeared to fascinate the team. However, during this placement, my fiancé had become pregnant and I was about to move to a new house to support her. This was an extra challenge to manage on top of studying and attending placement. As much as I was excited to go through placement, deep down I wanted to get through it swiftly. I did not discuss my concerns of balancing commitments with any staff at university. However, most of them knew my circumstances as a student who was adjusting to the prospect of being a parent. I had informed the placement educator in an introductory email that I was dyslexic and required reasonable adjustments; I wanted to prompt my educator to integrate enabling learning styles to support my develop-ment on placement. This didn't occur. But, despite being riddled with impostor syndrome from the start of the course and during placement, I was determined to do well and pass the placement outcomes, just like everyone else in my cohort.

On my first day, I spent time with my educator, shadowing her clin-ical appointments.

On my first week, my educator threw me into the deep end and suggested that I take the lead for the next appointment. Unprepared, I felt nervous and under pressure, almost as if I was being set up to fail. However, I took the challenge and saw it as a learning opportunity. I understood that she would be assessing me but it would have been kind to inform me that she would be assessing my communication skills with the client. I felt that in the feedback she provided to me, she did not give an accurate assessment of my communication skills. She perceived difficulties in my body language, eye contact and use of words, which I openly and respectfully disagreed with. It seemed as if that the char-acteristics of my personhood were not the norm in this profession. As a student, I took on board her analysis, but I felt on edge, not knowing when the next 'hidden assessment' would be.

Throughout the practice placement I did my best to maintain a proactive approach in my learning, seeking learning opportunities from different clinicians on the days my educator wasn't in. Despite this, I felt like her personal assistant, delegated to do clerical duties. Although I learned about administrative duties, it felt as if no other option was up for discussion because the educator did not trust me. Additionally, as a dyslexic student, my biggest challenge involved being efficient in writing clinical notes, as I had highlighted in my introductory email and outlined on my SWOT analysis, which was also submitted to my educator. On one occasion, I completed clinical notes from a visit to the hot-desking office room, a working environment filled with clinicians. When my educator read my clinical notes, she called me over to her desk, then suddenly she critiqued the notes, audibly in the open office, expressing negative remarks. Some clinicians in the office visibly shook their heads in sheer embarrassment. I was humiliated, my confidence took a hit, my fear of failure magnified, and impostor phenomenon intensified.

I felt pressure to work harder, but the more I tried, the less positive affirmation I received from my educator. As a student, I understood the influence my educator yielded in determining the progress and outcome of the placement – the power was firmly in her hands. As a Black person, I felt disempowered to speak out and feel heard in the placement, due to frequent incidents of *over scrutiny and assumptions* from my educator. Throughout the practice placement other similar incidents occurred and after the halfway point, a dyslexia specialist from the university came to provide support. However, all it did was negatively compound my learning experience, adding further pressure, making me feel *an easy target*. I felt this person brought in from the university to help was more invested in maintaining a good relationship with the clinicians for future students who may be allocated a placement. Any concerns I raised were dismissed. The university representative reiterated the importance of maintaining good relationships with educators, despite so much effort I was already putting into this.

Two weeks before the end of the placement, I was informed that the outcome of placement was a referral. Shock, denial and anger ensued. My approach as a student is always to be respectful, honest and diligent. Despite disclosing information about my learning difficulty and *pleading for patience*, I was never allowed the adjustments to fully enable me in the placement. I had the opportunity to appeal the outcome of placement, but I did not take up that option. I felt let down by the university. My voice was silenced. I had no other option but to go with the decision.

I reflected on this experience through a critical race lens. I see I was over scrutinised and given additional challenges because I had shared my learning difficulties which intersected with my *exoticised* Black identity, and these came together to disadvantage me on this placement (Crenshaw 2016).

Brief analysis of the placements

For the three authors, three main themes were identified from the case stories of placement: microaggressions, disempowerment and a lack of a sense of belonging.

Microaggressions

A common theme that was identified throughout the placements was the use of microaggressions. According to Sue *et al.* (2007a, 2007b), racial microaggressions relate to the specific behaviours, destructive attitudes, jokes and humiliations that persons racialised as BAME face daily. Moreover Sue *et al.* (2007a, 2007b) refers to microaggressions as the new face of racism and categorises them into:

- microassaults – overt racial behaviours or acts, non-verbal and verbal discrimination designed to intentionally offend and hurt an individual (Proctor *et al.* 2016)

- microinsults – as a contrast to microassaults, these present as more subtle acts that might be considered as disrespectful, insensitive or exclusionary (Proctor *et al.* 2016)

- microinvalidations – communications that do not appreciate the daily difficulties BAME individuals have to experience in everyday life (Proctor *et al.* 2016).

Hammond *et al.*'s (2019) study identified some key examples of microaggressions, including avoiding eye contact, physically touching hair, and asking 'where are you *really* from?' What is evident from this study is that racial microaggressions are not only displayed by practice educators but often also by the wider team and even service users. This links to a broader issue of BAME heritage students experiencing outcomes due to continued institutional racism in health and social care (Hammond *et al.* 2019). Microaggressions may not always be intentional but derive from learned ideology. Microaggression is, for the authors, another label for just institutionally emboldened racism. However, as there is very limited literature and research of the experiences of BAME populations of occupational therapy students on placement, this is an area that needs addressing and research to support a strategized approach informed by critical race studies to enable justice and equity for students on placement.

Disempowerment

Throughout the above placement experiences, there is a reluctance to challenge any forms of injustice due to racism concerns for fear of being labelled as a *troublemaker* or a *problematic student*. For any student racialised as BAME, not being empowered to raise concerns of racism creates real fear that merely discussing these specific issues that need addressing will lead to the practice educator failing them unjustly. This is supported by a study conducted by Hammond *et al.* (2019) where students felt that microaggressions had a significant impact on their success. For example, for many BAME heritage students there is a perception that there are lower or higher expectations of them, and they feel that they are required to prove themselves more than their white counterparts (Hammond *et al.* 2019). Therefore, challenging microaggressions may present as counterproductive as they don't necessarily want to appear difficult. However, the study conducted by Hammond *et al.* (2019) related to physiotherapy students in the UK and their experiences. While physiotherapy is a separate profession to occupational therapy, both professions are governed by the Health and Care Professions Council and the study is therefore relatable to occupational therapy students. Hence, not being empowered and afforded agency to complain to bring about change in the system is detrimental to the students, not enabling them to be their whole self on placements or the course and feel that they belong in the institution.

Belonging

Research highlights the importance of one having a sense of belonging, as it positively impacts an individual's academic success and motivation

(Freeman *et al.* 2007). According to Palmer and Maramba (2015), racial microaggressions can have a significant impact on a student's sense of belonging. Therefore, for ALL students to have a positive university experience and eventually graduate, the support given to students must be personalized, and not standardized, to ensure a sense of belonging. However, according to University College London (UCL) (2020), students of BAME heritage backgrounds have reported having a lower sense of belonging compared to their white counterparts. A running theme throughout each experience was the lack of adequate support when experiencing racial microaggressions. As it stands, many BAME racialised occupational therapy students are required to overcome these issues in isolation and are unable to openly communicate their concerns, which often impacts their mental health (Torres *et al.* 2010). Moreover, Palmer and Maramba (2015) explain that the significant impact on BAME students' sense of belonging can intensify emotional exhaustion, increasing the prospect of students withdrawing from their course. This therefore suggests that the racial microaggressions experienced by BAME racialised occupational therapy students could be directly affecting them in completing their occupational therapy course.

What is evident is that if the issues around racial microaggressions and racial equality are not addressed, in the long term it will have negative implications on experiences for students from BAME heritage backgrounds, and create increased barriers between occupational therapy professionals and patients. Ultimately, this will have undesirable consequences on the occupational therapy profession. In addition to this, students from BAME heritage backgrounds have expressed the lack of diversity in higher education institutions – this includes a lack of representation of lecturers and practice educators who are of BAME backgrounds (Batty 2019). Hodge and Marsh (2015) express this as a major problem as there has been a severe shortage of professionals representing BAME backgrounds in every level of education – and as a result, student engagement is affected due to a lack of role and real models.

All of these points lead us to a perpetual lack of representation of people from BAME heritages in occupational therapy education and maintains the status quo of institutional racism in these institutions. Representation matters and disrupts the status quo of racism through enabling diverse ideas, creations and innovations to be heard, actioned and embedded, which creates a more successful and happier organisation. The organisation becomes less comfortable with living with the power and privilege imbalances created by homogeneity and dominating groups (Rock & Grant 2016; Rock *et al.* 2016).

A few suggestions listed to mitigate injustices and create an equitable learning experience for students racialised as BAME

- Improve the racial literacy of all stakeholders involved with occupational therapy students – this includes students and educators too. This will enable, as a starter, everyone to have access to the same language so the concerns raised are understood in the context in which they are raised. For example, cultural competency is a corporate diversity tick-box exercise and has shown to not change institutional racism (Dobbin & Kalev 2018). Whereas, cultural humility is ongoing learning to improve racial literacy, to add to knowledge, to keep checking in on yourself and your actions to perpetuate antiracism, equity and justice stance.

- Make sure policies, processes and culture enable the investigation and addressing of incidents of racism that are raised. Have an incident log-book to document racism incidents raised and outcomes, because, as discussed, accumulative stress from everyday racism can lead to ill-health (Gee & Ford 2011; Stanley *et al.* 2019).

- Provide spaces where the students racialised as BAME can share experiences without judgement and fear, where they are heard by people in positions of power and they see impactful outcomes, individual or institutional, from their racialised trauma being valued and being fuel for change-making. At London South Bank University, Musharrat is a convener of two affinity groups in allied health professions: the Race and Cultural Equity Group for students and staff who identify as racialised as BAME, and an Allyship and Cultural Equity Group for students and staff who identify as white. The focus of both the groups is equity and justice in the curricula and they can feed back to management and executives when relevant. They are safe but active spaces that remove the hierarchy of power between student and teacher to improve the feelings of belonging, and humanise relationships.

- Create a support and sharing group space for educators who identify as racialised as BAME.

- Facilitate the development of positive teacher-student relationships, which has been proven to enhance a student's sense of belonging (Burke *et al.* 2016).

- Expose students to positive role and real models from the Black and minoritised communities (Arday 2015; Dhanda 2009).

- Host inclusive events from the offset. Thomas *et al.* (2017) suggest that belonging begins at induction, presenting a 'logic chain' linking induction activities to student retention and success. In the United States, Duke University's occupational therapy doctorate programme has a recruitment and retention staff member from BIPOC heritage, dedicated to retention and support of minoritised students. This is not to create difference but to provide tailored support for equity.

- (For universities) Develop mentorship programmes gathering a pool of clinicians from BAME heritage backgrounds for students from the same heritage backgrounds (culture match is critical) and pay the mentors for their time. The Coalition of Occupational Therapy Advocates for Diversity (COTAD) offers this programme, although the mentors are volunteers and not affiliated with any occupational therapy programmes and neither are the students.

A word of caution though, do not burden your students and staff who identify as racialised as BAME to do the work for change alone – it is the responsibility of all to disrupt racism and create a just and equitable environment for learning, as this will benefit everyone, especially students and teachers, and hence benefit the members of the public with whom occupational therapy graduates work.

Conclusion

Based on the authors' previous experiences as students, they believe, and the evidence is showing this too, that the profession still has a way to go to eradicate racism and to establish ways to effectively support students, educators and occupational therapists who identify as racialized as BAME. One of the main issues with racism is that the burden of proof lies with the victim of racism, therefore they feel that it is more stress on top of the experience of racism and so usually no action is taken. The approach institutionally should be to change the environment so that in leadership, strategies, principles, policies, practices and culture it is always structurally framed on being antiracist, just and equitable.

Reflective quadrant: Identifying, recording and understanding learning from the chapter

What? (Describe what have I learnt)

Relevance? (Why is this topic relevant to me/to my practice? Relate/align to/with, e.g., research literature, professional bodies' proficiencies/competencies, service delivery/service user benefit, legislation – briefly and critically discuss)

How will this learning change me/my practice?

What actions do I have to follow up on to develop my learning in this area or apply to my practice? (SMART goal format or similar)

Ethnic Neutral Occupational Therapy Services in Health and Social Care Contribute to Maintaining Structural Inequity

Musharrat J. Ahmed-Landeryou, Peter Bredu-Darkwa

Introduction

This chapter aims to critically explore the history and current consequences of ethnic neutrality (ethnocentric) in occupational therapy practice and services. The chapter calls the occupational therapy community in to interrogate its own house when it comes to antiracist approach to service transformation. As political activist Steve Biko (Stubbs 1978: 92) stated in his book, *I Write What I Like*: 'The most potent weapon of the oppressor is the mind of the oppressed.' We must change ourselves, our minds first, understand how we contribute/sustain racism in systems, before we go to create change.

Thus, the critical questions that guide this chapter are:

- How can occupational therapy deliver an antiracist and equitable service?

- How does the profession stop recycling the white supremacy construct of occupational therapy practice globally?

Background

Occupational therapy is part of the health and social care system and built on the core principles of person-centredness and social justice (Duncan 2020). Occupational therapists treat the whole person, using the modality of activities as treatment, regardless of the impairment, and in doing so are aware of all the environments impacting on the whole person, such as culture, politics and welfare system (Black & Wells 2007; Cole & Tufano 2020). Occupational therapists must be careful not to overlay their values, culture or judgement, to enable person-centred practice, and deliver a service that treats people with dignity and respect (Black & Wells 2007; Duncan 2020). Therefore, therapists must critically examine and be aware of how knowledge, education, policies, practices and processes and their own biases shape service delivery in their attempt to be individualised and authentically culturally responsive to service users. Inherently, occupational therapy is ethnically neutral, as its history, philosophy, theories and education are built on Eurocentric constructs and white supremacy ideology.

Ethnic neutrality in medicine is recognised as inherently enabling othering, and disregarding the necessity of diversity, inclusion and equity within its various organisations, services and disciplines (Keshet & Popper-Giveon 2017). Ethnic neutrality perpetuates institutional racism. The framework of neutrality may still enable some staff of BME heritages in the profession; however, it is not able to reconcile the inequalities and inequities that staff and service users of BME backgrounds experience in health and social care organisations or services (Keshet & Popper-Giveon 2017). This privilege perception and behaviour in medicine can also be named as the superiority complex of Eurocentrism (Saini 2019). It is based on the socially constructed concept of race, so that colonisers could justify the harm and oppression caused to indigenous/minoritised people or nations, and the subsequent controlling of native/indigenous people for economic gain. Professor Jane Elliot (2020) says repeatedly that 'there is one race, the human race', and that 'human beings created racism and learnt to be racist and hence can unlearn it'. Saini (2019) adds that it is not simple to unlearn racism and undo the dominance of Eurocentrism, because those that benefit and profit from it do not want to give it up; that is, equality and equity are perceived as the loss of privilege for those with power.

The founders of occupational therapy were racialised as white and were from the United States, UK and Canada. The cultural norms for occupational therapy in health and social care in these countries were from a white supremacy ideology, and the philosophy, processes and practices are still dominated by Eurocentricism (Pentland & Pentland

2015; Andersen & Reed 2017; Perryman-Fox & Cox 2020). Occupational therapy leaders, clinicians and educators carry on the white hegemony of the profession because it enables them to continue the teachings and principles of delivering services based on the knowledge of the Global North (Europe, North Americas) (Grenier 2020; Picower 2009). It has taken occupational therapy 104 years to use the term racism and recognise that racism exists (Kronenberg 2021b).

This may be a reason why there is a trend to decolonising the curriculum because the knowledge being recycled in university education is dominated by the Global North – that is, western-centric colonial origins framing the knowledge (Bhambra *et al.* 2018; Grenier 2020). The message the current occupational therapy curriculum content sends is that the knowledge that is worthy is that from the Global North, and this pushes to the margins, hides and devalues Global South and indigenous knowledges (Freire 1993; Dei 1996; Bhambra *et al.* 2018). Decolonising the curriculum is trying to provide equal space for knowledges from the Global South and North by centring co-design of curriculum with the very populations that are marginalised, discriminated and oppressed (Decolonising SOAS Working Group 2018; Ahmed 2020; Liyanage 2020).

So, you may be wondering about the relevance of all this to occupational therapy practice and services in relation to ethnic neutrality. We posit that if universities are delivering knowledge dominated from the Global North, and occupational therapy is taught at university, then occupational therapy philosophy, concepts, processes and research are also framed by the knowledge of the Global North, which graduates then recycle into practice. This will not promote antiracism explicitly and will constrain equity (Keshet & Popper-Giveon 2017), and is not true to imbuing the philosophy and principles of social justice and person centredness through occupational therapy practice and processes.

This further highlights the need to take a critical look at the various education and training of occupational therapy practitioners as approved by the World Federation of Occupational Therapists (WFOT) (2016) in relation to what services are delivering. This then draws attention to critically review the WFOT as it is sanctioning a 'regime' of a white centric way of teaching occupational therapy that has been transferred worldwide. This is sanctioned through governance structures in the WFOT, governance being a 'framework of authority and accountability that defines and controls the outputs, outcomes and benefits from projects, programmes, and portfolios' (Association for Project Management 2022). So, for the WFOT to disrupt this recycling, it will require acknowledgement from the WFOT that this is happening as a contributory factor of the organisation, and then for the WFOT to reflect, review, reframe and rebuild itself to be decentred from whiteness before strategising the support of antiracism and anti-discrimination as explicit actions that need to be demonstrated by institutes seeking approval of occupational therapy programmes by the WFOT. The WFOT and other affiliate national bodies should be thinking of directionality in the development of culturally responsive educational and training programmes. Currently, many of the core texts are predominantly authored by individuals racialised as white, so even if they write about culture, it will be from a white lens, providing narrowed diversity and inclusion perspectives. Developing culturally responsive occupational therapy service starts with education, which should centre lecturers, research and literature with a breadth of staff and authors from Global South heritage to disrupt the dominance of Eurocentrism.

Critical question: How can occupational therapy services deliver antiracist and equitable services?

To start with, the profession must take a critical look at the theoretical basis of our interventions and delivery of services. While occupational therapy theories, models and frames of reference from the western world offer much insight into the practice and services delivery of occupational therapy, those who receive these services, and practitioners, need ways to make sense of these theories and models that better align meaningfully and impactfully with the lived experiences of service users. Occupational therapy services providers must therefore enable effective, relevant and satisfactory culturally integrated provision to make services equitably fit for purpose (Acheson & Schneider-Bean 2019). The services must be fit for the service users from minoritised populations if they are to meet their person-centred needs.

This is enabled by practitioners, and thus educators with their students, by having to engage continually in improving their racial and cultural literacy to show they are invested in disrupting ethnic neutrality and racism in health and social care. Educators and researchers must make efforts to facilitate occupational therapy theories and models to be culturally responsive and accessible, and more applicable to the lived experiences of the minoritised populations, not centring those that racialise as white or from the Global North. This will improve the skills and competencies of students, and prepare them to work with service users from minoritised populations, who may have societal values and cultural contexts different from them and the dominating western-centric ideology (Shirley 2016). This should enable occupational therapy students and those who graduate to qualified practitioners to develop services that are culturally responsive and provide equity. This also enables organisations to promote inclusion, and disrupt exclusion and othering to meet the needs of the local populations and individuals they work with (Salvan 2013).

Adopting a pluriverse cultural approach to occupational therapy services

Culture is 'the conscious and unconscious content that a group learns, shares, and transmits from generation to generation that organises life and helps interpret existence' (Diller 2015: 172). It represents larger modal behaviour patterns and social tendencies of groups of people, and features in the practices individuals and communities are seen to embody (Iwama 2004). Culture is a social construct and complex; it is a system that comprises many different parts, which dynamically interact with each other. It includes components such as history, values, local politics, communication style, beliefs and practices and more (Diller 2015), which must be well understood and appreciated, so that therapists are familiar, have understanding, and are able to integrate it in practice. In ensuring that service delivery relates to individual service users, is person-centred and enables the best of outcomes for them, practitioners must demonstrate competent understanding of the complexity of culture in health and wellbeing. Culture is fundamental for occupational therapy as it can elucidate the day-to-day realities for minoritised and marginalised service users and therapists (Iwama 2007). Hence a pluriverse cultural approach centres the person's and their community's cultures, denotes that culture is not homogeneous, and affords many opportunities to direct person-centred transformations that can be cultivated from occupational therapy.

Iwama (2007) cautioned that there is little emphasis from the profession on inward reflection on the cultural construction of occupational therapy, to understand how it is propagating exclusion and othering of individuals and communities that are minoritised and marginalised. Hence the profession must interrogate how occupational therapy is maintaining the status quo of institutional racism through its knowledge, training, practice and service delivery. By starting to do this, the profession will then develop learning on how to disrupt delivering ethnic neutral services, and be antiracist and hence equitable in provision. This will only help grow the profession towards improving cultural responsibility and not only promote but enact delivering equitable services. Cultural responsibility is the duty of governments, organisations and individuals to be respectful of the mix of different cultural manifestations within their societies to safeguard the human rights of people (UNESCO 2003). We may need to re-examine and reframe our frameworks, models and theories of practice, and explicitly situate antiracism and equity within them. Practitioners must administer interventions that service users can culturally relate to (Iwama 2007) and feel safe with (UNESCO 2003), by centring the person not only as a doing being, but a cultural body that belongs within a community. This can only serve to improve the person-centred relevance and reliability of the therapy, which may motivate individuals to participate in interventions essential for the service user's self-identified transformation, recovery and wellbeing.

Discriminatory treatment in hospitals because of a person's inability to feel culturally safe and relate to treatment interventions and modalities can lead to further harming the person and, in some cases, to their death (Acheson & Schneider-Bean 2019). This leads to a denial of health and wellbeing due to the 'reduced' quality of healthcare service delivery. Ignoring the necessity to integrate culture in the delivery of occupational therapy reinforces a particularly negative view of the value of culture, and that occupational therapy is for the privileged few – which runs counter to its principles of person-centredness and occupational justice (Córdoba 2020). The insistence on the use of the western lens on service delivery, without recourse to individualised culturally based values, undermines service users' sense of being and belonging, which are vital elements of occupational justice (Lopez-Littleton *et al.* 2018). Guajardo Córdoba (2020) stressed how occupational therapy through its westernised ideologies has caused occupational justice to become a new form of epistemic and cognitive colonisation of the profession, which operates under universalist, essentialist, liberal assumptions, typical of modern western rationality. Westernisation here suggests the adoption of European culture with regards to mentality, education, training and healthcare service delivery (Thong 2012). When we do not have services that are culturally responsive and responsible then health and social care services start to harm populations. For example, in the UK in the East London boroughs, South Asian women have 65 per cent more likelihood of dying early from heart disease when compared to the general population trend; and people from Bangladeshi and Pakistani communities are 'five or six times more likely to have type 2 diabetes than the general population' (Reza & van Heel 2022). Reza and van Heel (2022) state that not all the reasons for the health disparities for this population have been figured out, but one aspect that needs addressing in the interventions and services is culture. Furthermore, in the United States, effective services that are culturally responsive and responsible use the term cultural respect and make culture integral to service delivery as it is critical to reducing health disparities and improves access to quality person-centred care (National Institutes of Health 2021).

The scope of the idea of occupational therapy service delivery and its colonial implications has no limits. The idea of justice during service delivery is proposed based on an ethical, political and cultural criterion (Córdoba 2020). The service delivery of occupational therapy is centred currently on the Eurocentric model of practice and fails to recognize other cultural forms of knowledge, beliefs and practices (DaCunha 2016). This means practice of occupational therapy has focused on European culture as expressed in various training curricula to the exclusion of a wider view of the indigenous people. To help improve occupational therapy service delivery in various cultural jurisdictions, colonialism of healthcare delivery must subside, and multiculturalism must rise. Academic and professional programmes need to purposefully include discussions of individualised and community culturally based values. This strategy will begin to prepare future therapists to thoughtfully engage in in-depth dialogues around culture, beliefs, practices and values systems and how they influence quality healthcare delivery.

Samson (2018) elucidates that the consequence of ignoring cultural difference in health is that indigenous patients can face systemic barriers in accessing medical services, including discrimination and racism. Failure of the profession to recognise individualised and community cultural values, beliefs and practices reinforces the status quo of institutional racism and leads to inequity and eventually poor outcomes for individuals and communities.

Training in cultural humility for occupational therapy practitioners

Cultural humility was originally conceived as a framework from which to educate United States medics in how to work with patients from a diversity of racial, ethnic and cultural heritages/backgrounds (Yeager & Bauer-Wu 2013). Cultural humility 'is a lifelong process of self-reflection and self-critique whereby the individual not only learns about another's culture, but one starts with an examination of her/his own beliefs and cultural identities' (Tervalon & Murray-Garcia 1998 cited in Yeager and Bauer-Wu 2013: 2). Hence the act of cultural humility is not an end point, but an ongoing invested engagement in lifelong learning, in critical consciousness in identifying and understanding explicitly your own biases and how your own upbringing and social environment has shaped your outlook and behaviours – and doing this in collaboration with service users, communities and peers (Kumagai & Lypson 2009). It has to be lifelong because culture is dynamic and is influenced by context, for example chronology, individuals, community, where in the globe you are, politics, economics and more (Yeager & Bauer-Wu 2013).

The lifelong concept fits well with occupational therapy because in training, and when qualified, all therapists must be able to demonstrate engagement in continuing reflective practice to improve their critical knowledge and understanding of current practice (Boyt Schell & Schell 2017). Also, they must be able to evidence reflective practice in line with registrable bodies' requirements (e.g. Health and Care Professions Council 2021). Engagement in cultural humility also enables the therapist to recognise the role of power, politics and privilege in health and social care provision (Agner 2020).

Cultural competency is typically defined as the skills that a clinician can employ to understand the cultural values, attitudes and behaviours of patients, especially those whose cultural background differs from that of the professional (Schouler-Ocak *et al.* 2015). Beagan (2018) outlines several ideas beyond cultural competencies that can be included for training staff:

- Cultural awareness or cultural sensitivity – being aware that cultural differences and similarities between people exist without assigning them to negative and positive values, better or worse, right or wrong (Dabbah 2014).

- Cultural responsivity – not just developing one's knowledge and understanding of various cultures but expanding the ways in which one thinks about the various dimensions of culture and how this shapes professional practice (Sullivan & A'Vant 2009).

- Cultural relevance – thinking about the skills required for practising in multicultural settings (Scherff & Spector 2011).

Cultural humility is moving on from cultural competence, as the latter assumes that culture is a finite and not a dynamic construct (Agner 2020). A study of 829 companies over 31 years (Dobbin *et al.* 2007: 26) identified that diversity training, for example cultural competency, showed 'no positive effects in the average workplace' and '[in] firms where training is mandatory or emphasizes the threat of lawsuits, training actually has negative effects on management diversity'. The study found that equality and diversity departments in organisations spent millions on purchasing these training schemes, yet the attitudes of the employees and the diversity of staff remained the same after training (Dobbin *et al.* 2007). Fundamentally for the organisations and the staff, these trainings become a tick-box exercise to meet metrics (Bregman 2012), placing a sticking plaster 'on a longstanding festering infected wound', which is a temporary solution, rather than the harder work of changing the structural issues, and leads to outcomes of inequity and institutional racism.

In essence, cultural humility training did start off as training for white practitioners or practitioners for whom it is not the norm to recognise the power imbalance, but it did not then take it further to actively train people to disrupt this imbalance. It's important to disrupt the European and western cultural dominance in the practice and service delivery of occupational therapy, and to focus on practice that is individualised, culturally based and co-produced with the people with whom the service works. A classic example of western dominance of practice can be observed in paediatric developmental milestones, which form the basis of most of our paediatric assessments and remain firmly aligned with traditional western child-rearing philosophies. According to Razack (1995), the assumption is that if these inadequacies could somehow be considered, especially in healthcare services, the impact of inequalities and inequities would reduce, which would include the practice of occupational therapists all over the world.

One of the authors of this chapter is from an African country, and he notes that occupational therapy in most African countries was designed by and for those racialised as white, western and middle class. Occupation-based treatments, therefore, reflect those sanctioned by white, middle-class society to reintegrate patients back into regular white society (Kiepek & Beagen 2018). This approach is what has been transferred to therapists from different continents and cultures and it fails to recognise the administration of individualised culturally based co-produced service delivery. It is important for the stakeholders in the design and accreditation of occupational therapy, services and curricula to recognise that cultural beliefs, values and practices may be relevant in some situations and contexts but not in others. There is therefore the need to increase support for critical and structural frameworks within education and healthcare contexts, which support this radical shift in knowledge structures to respect cultural values and diversity in practices when with service users. The Canadian Association of Occupational Therapists (CAOT) (2011), in its position statement on cultural safety, states that all delivering occupational therapy (i.e. educators, preceptors and mentors) should critically examine the approaches to diversity, which includes people's cultures, and how these are being conveyed to learners, to ensure they attend to biases embedded in the profession and professional education, power relations between clients and therapists and within the profession, and connections between individual experiences and broader social power relations.

Training regarding cultural aspects at institutional, service and individual levels should be an ongoing endeavour for continuous development, as society changes and its understanding of communities is more informed. Applying cultural humility training in occupational therapy curricula and practice provides an active learning process – a process to unravel the endemic institutional issues and unlearn the western centric dominance of practice. We urgently need trained practitioners to start to disrupt the status quo of ethnic neutrality of service delivery, so that service users feel safe to come to occupational therapy services for their recovery, and employees feel safe in carrying out their work.

Creating culturally equitable service delivery

Embedding cultural humility and disruption actions is a lifestyle change for occupational therapy services. It involves designing services from an equity and justice lens (e.g. inclusivity, intersectionality, sexuality and socio-economic factors, among others), disrupting the status quo by building culturally responsive and responsible services on a foundation of more truthful histories, and fostering an appreciation of the people of the community. It is necessary for practitioners and occupational therapy students to go through three levels of awareness during their training and when transitioning into the practice world. These are self-awareness, social awareness and global awareness (DaCunha 2016). It is during these levels that students and entry-level practitioners acknowledge the diversity of the world they live within. First, self-awareness focuses on exploration and evaluation of yourself to obtain a sense of cultural, self and social identity. Second, social awareness stresses the need to understand the societal functions and attempt to analyse the issues in your community and cultural context. Third is global awareness, which encourages you to practise critical reflection and to empathize with the struggles and oppression of others within the world they practise. DaCunha's levels are necessary if you don't already have this level of conscientisation as the norm; many indigenous nations already have this way of being embedded.

Various theoretical assumptions, for example the model of human occupation (MOHO), stress service users' motivation as being a critical and vital part of participation in treatment programmes and interventions. Integrating and respecting differences in culture and values will improve the motivation of the individual, which plays an important part in therapy. Also, acknowledging the differences in culture, values and practices of service users will guide practitioners towards improving their acceptance of other cultures, by actively applying cultural humility. This awareness is specifically for occupational therapy practitioners whose core principles are built on an understanding of culture, diversity, person-centredness and justice; through their curiosity and the information provided, they will then be able to acquire the motivation to use their path of self-development in the delivery of occupational therapy services. The profession should be trained and have skills to create a balance of how and why practitioners can adapt their services to different cultures in practice. Training guides and curricula must integrate knowledge from the Global South, and the best practices from these places must meld into the curricula to showcase the Global South and the knowledges and practices that enable their communities to thrive. Not only should a practitioner view the world from other cultures' perspectives, but the practitioner should also be able to adapt to the way of life of the various cultures by adjusting their own perspectives, behaviours and attitudes (Keshet & Popper-Giveon 2017).

The current occupational therapy regime is a practice where Eurocentrism dominates, where a certain group of individuals is superior, and others inferior, where there is denial and lack of recognition of the different therapeutic approaches needed to work with individuals from a diversity of cultures from the Global South, and the Global South in the Global North. Creating opportunities for practitioners to move easily in and out of different cultural worldviews is necessary in their duty to cause no harm. Practitioners must accept that, even though they may not agree with other cultures, they need to employ a pluriverse cultural approach for relevant, relatable, safe, effective and quality delivery of service. Occupational therapy services must respect the beliefs and values of individuals and communities from BME backgrounds and understand them from the person's or group's cultural perspectives.

Existing occupational therapy culture has not yet fully articulated diverse worldviews that are not understood using western centrism, regarding occupation, health and wellbeing, and the link between them. Taking into consideration the diversity of the global world, incorporating different worldviews would be a valuable contribution to expanding the relevance of occupational therapy (Iwama 2007).

Critical question: How does the profession stop recycling the white lens construct of occupational therapy practice globally?

It has to be a multifactorial approach, because for occupational therapy students, staff and educators to stop recycling the status quo of whiteness, the construct, in its philosophy, practices and education, is a wicked problem. Rittel and Webber (1973) identified the term 'a wicked problem' – a problem that is difficult to define, a societal problem that has multiple components, and these components are constantly shifting and reconfiguring. They say there is not an optimal solution to a wicked problem, but a solution that is good enough for right now, for the current context. The solution found and applied will need reviewing, reframing and rebuilding to remain contextual in line with societal changes and trends, politics, laws and evidence base (Rittel & Webber 1973). We could restate the whiteness construct in the occupational therapy profession as Eurocentricism which is contributing to ethnic neutral service delivery.

Roger Kline's (2020) article, 'After the speeches: What now for NHS staff race discrimination?', could provide a way to strategise disruption to the status quo of recycling ethnic neutral occupational therapy service delivery. Kline's (2020) article sets out ten points for what needs to be in place from 'board to ward' to demonstrate authentic commitment to change.

1. Antiracism, inclusion, diversity and equity must be core for boards and should be a permanent item on the agenda for business

In occupational therapy, no board and its members should be set up without its members articulating and signing up clearly to a commitment to antiracism, anti-discrimination and anti-oppression. Also, the boards must ensure that they have a roadmap, a strategy of how they are going to action, monitor, measure and revaluate this cyclically, and be explicit about timelines. Occupational therapy professional bodies (e.g. Royal College of Occupational Therapists (UK), American Occupational Therapy Association (United States), Associacao Brasileira dos Terapeutas Ocupacionais (Brazil)), and organisations that regulate the profession (e.g. Health and Care Professions Council (UK), National Board for Certification in Occupational Therapy (United States), Ministério da Saúde and Ministério da Educação (Brazil)) currently do not practise this. None have made acknowledgement that institutional racism exists in their organisations, and only one is known to the authors (Royal College of Occupational Therapists) to have started the journey to actively reject racism and actively challenge and remove it from the profession.

2. Occupational therapy organisations must pause, and review, refocus and rebuild

First, all occupational therapy professional bodies and regulators need to collect accurate data regarding members and registrants. This will enable them to see the diversity of representation of their members and registrants, which will enable them to start identifying trends and potential areas to further investigate. Kline (2020) says boards must stop being not open about their equality data and lack of proactiveness. Diversity in the student and staff populations of occupational therapy will only benefit the profession and the people they work with because it will: enable better understanding of difference; celebrate difference and enable belonging; create a safe and open team working; enable better decision-making and promote creative and innovative thinking; enable staff and service users to be treated with dignity and respect; and provide a fair, accessible and therefore better service to a diverse population because the service will not be built on a Eurocentric foundation (Matebeni 2012; Dike 2013: Marder 2017; Chartered Institute of Personnel and Development 2020). It's not just about representation.

3. Occupational therapy boards and services should sign actions that are evidence based to enable delivery of ethnorelative services

Boards and services should have clear action plans that relate to strategies and measures that are disrupting the status quo of institutional racism, decolonising education, developing ethnorelative theories, principles and practices. Ethnorelative means transitioning through acceptance that there are differences, then adapting to get ready to change and finally integrating principles of diversity, equality and equity to begin the process of change (Hammer *et al.* 2003). When this is applied to occupational therapy services, practices and processes, it will enable staff to deliver culturally responsive services.

4. Occupational therapy leaders, boards and services must be proactive, prepared and preventative

There needs to be full current data that enables understanding of the trend and performance of services and examines and scrutinizes what is working and improves what is not. There must be examination of where it needs improving; there must be clear purpose, strategy and accountability. As stated, an ethnorelative strategy must be embedded, to enable disrupting the recycling of racism and health inequities and the white construct of occupational therapy services. This will start to disrupt the white construct of health and social care. But for this to happen, it must start with occupational therapy education; it must be role-modelled by the professional bodies and regulators.

5. Accountability needs to be embedded

The starting point for any health or social care service, ergo occupational therapy, should be responsibility – taking the responsibility to make sure services are culturally responsive and responsible, enabling belonging and equity, by applying values-based and strengths-based frameworks (Davis 2016). Accountability raises its head when responsibility has failed. But metrics can hold services, organisations, managers and staff to account by setting meaningful goals that are time limited and understood by all to enable buy-in and engagement (Kline 2020). This is from recruitment through to delivery, and from board to frontline, of the occupational therapy services.

6. Organisations cannot be diverse and inclusive, and services ethnorelative, without environmental psychological safety

It is well known that if you experience racism, discrimination, bullying or harassment at work, you do not perform at your fullest abilities and you do not feel wellbeing at work, and hence sick days are often taken (Williams *et al.* 2019; Hewett *et al.* 2018). Boards and leaders must put in place policies, strategies, resources and training to create an environment of psychological safety for the wellbeing of staff and for the benefit of service delivery for the service users (Edmonson & Roloff 2008; Rangachari & Woods 2020).

7. Occupational therapy professional bodies and regulators and leaders must be responsible role models

This is about culture, and the tone of that is set by the boards and leaders within organisations and within the profession. They have to make it a priority that services are ethnorelative, as the action and potential benefits are just and fair to disrupt racism and the health inequities status quo in health and social care. Most necessary is that these people are real models, that is genuine, accessible and relatable.

8. 'Equality, diversity and inclusion are drivers of service improvement.' This is everyone's business, not just a few allocated personnel (Kline 2020)

Do not roll out Black and minoritised individuals to lead, or showcase leadership, and carry the majority of the burden of antiracism change – especially when organisations do not share this group's presence in all the other top leadership roles consistently; for example, see the 'Snowy White Peaks' report (Kline 2014). These roles and the work must be allocated in the budgets and resourcing needs as usual practice.

9. Health and social care organisations and services must be supported and enabled

To disrupt ethnic neutral service delivery, services such as occupational therapy must actively join with the movements for equality, equity and antiracism. This will enable them to ally with groups that are doing the antiracism, anti-discrimination and anti-oppression work to better learn and understand what is needed to continuously develop and embed ethnorelative services. This will enable development of a 'national good practice repository on diversity and inclusion' which does not currently exist (Kline 2020) for occupational therapy.

10. There needs to be urgent national focus on antiracist practice, metrics and governance

Doing this will demonstrate process, outcomes and progress in disrupting institutional racism and hence build ethnorelative health and social care services. Every year, reports must be produced and published publicly showing what is happening with regard to antiracism and equity for service users and staff (e.g. the WRES 2020 from NHS England (2021)), and actions reported.

Conclusion

This chapter is a call to action to review occupational therapy governance boards for antiracist praxis. It is not enough to educate (and hope for humility in) privileged peoples in institutionally racist systems – in fact, it keeps things exactly as they are. What is needed are actions to disrupt the structures by making it matter to them (e.g. reputations, salary, opportunities), because when it matters to them it is then valued and becomes personal to mobilise change. Actions speak louder than platitudes. It is time for occupational therapy as a profession and all professional bodies, regulators, leaders, students, clinicians and educators of the profession to acknowledge institutional racism, and then consciously, and conscientiously, disrupt the status quo of ethnic neutral service delivery.

Starting practical steps:

- Care about making antiracist change on a personal level – make it matter to you and do some work on yourself.

- Start by improving the racial literacy of the staff.

- Review your service using a proactive culturally responsive/ responsible framework, then make actions and identify antiracism and equity measures for service evaluation and accountability.

- Give all staff antiracism training each year, making it developmental, and measure impact on service outcomes.

Reflective quadrant: Identifying, recording and understanding learning from the chapter

What? (Describe what have I learnt)	**Relevance?** (Why is this topic relevant to me/to my practice?) Relate/align to/with, e.g., research literature, professional bodies' proficiencies/competencies, service delivery/service user benefit, legislation – briefly and critically discuss)
How will this learning change me/my practice?	**What actions do I have to follow up on to develop my learning in this area or apply to my practice?** (SMART goal format or similar)

— CHAPTER 7 —

Antiracism as Means and Ends

Isla Emery-Whittington, Jaime Daniel Leite Junior, Sheela Ivlev

Introduction

The purpose of this chapter is unapologetically to further one of the goals of global racialised communities: ending racism. Farias *et al.* (2020: 243) explains that the 'racialisation of life and the production of racial inequality permeates the everyday life of all agents, whether those who suffer violence, whether those who practise and/or legitimise violence, or those who watch them'. Measuring antiracism is a small aspect but a necessary action of the antiracism approach, yet it does not follow that racism, with its roots in colonialism, is easily circumscribable or open to being scrutinised and grappled with. This chapter argues why and how measures of antiracism require nothing less than the collaborative strength of collectives using multiple strategies across multiple spheres of influence to bring transformation. We outline a stepwise antiracism programme that includes honest identification of sites of racism, bespoke and contextualised plans, in full and transparent collaboration with expert collectives. As antiracism and decolonisation are entirely contextual, we do not endorse standardised antiracism measures, closed protocols or universals. Thus, the critical question that guides this chapter is:

- How can we suggest possibilities for an antiracist praxis in occupational therapy, considering different contexts, breaking with an universalist approach?

Background

We bring together our experiences of building antiracist collectives from three different continents in this collaboration, which is more than text but the result of approximation and mutual learning, this itself is antiracism in action. One author is a cisgender, gay, Latino American man who lives in Brazil and was able to enter the public university due to the social policies of quotas, access and permanence. The other authors are cisgender, heterosexual women, one a first generation Bengali American and the other Māori, with responsibilities to her tribal community and Māori peer network. We each share a commitment to support the growing BIPOC occupational therapy global communities. We make reference to the acronym BIPOC (Black, Indigenous, People of Color); it is an imperfect term, and we acknowledge that experiences of oppression, exclusion and mistreatment are not the same for everyone, and attention and distinctions need contextualising. BIPOC is not a measure or a category (Sarfo-Annin 2020).

Two of the authors experience English as a second and third language. Although this text arrives to you in English, it was also thought and elaborated on in Brazilian Portuguese and Māori, thus requiring delicate translation of theorising from different languages and ideologies. This collaboration of thought and experience about occupational therapy, racism and its inevitable occupational impacts on everyday life is both a privilege and painful process of excavation. Each of the authors has undeservedly experienced racialised aggression in everyday life and overt racism while training, practising and/or researching occupational therapy. Therefore, writing to decolonize demands careful co-witness to racial trauma, co-theorizing possibilities and collectively transforming these into action. Together we resist, heal and transform the effects of racism, including founding DisruptOT global collective, Māori OT Network, Dona Ivone Lara Group, and many more collaboratives.

This chapter is purposefully written to collectives of antiracism champions, BIPOC colleagues and allies. We acknowledge your commitment, courage and strength. If your reader experience is about unlearning or recognising the need to share power, we commend these steps and encourage the next antiracist actions. The following is not meant for those just beginning their antiracism journey. It is written for those prepared to fight for their own and our collective liberation.

Defining racism and antiracism

Measuring antiracism requires identification of both the obvious and hidden aspects of racism. Racism is wielded at systems, at relational and internal levels of human experience. Racist systems, structures and policies ensure access to material resources and power, and opportunities are unfairly distributed to benefit some and exclude others (Almeida 2018; Williams & Mohammed 2013). Interpersonal racism refers to relationships and interactions between people that may include violence, expressions of hostility, surveillance, refusal to act, fragility and microaggressions. Internalised racism refers to the belief in and identification with negative stereotypes and assessments of one's culture by a dominant culture, that can lead to self-loathing and accelerated ageing (Geronimus *et al.* 2006).

Race as a biological truth has long been disproven (American Anthropological Association 1998). As it is an entirely social invention then, critical scholars and activists question the societal context within which people are actively taught to perceive 'race' (Munanga & Gomes 2016; Wilkerson 2020) and practise racism. Interpreting differences positively or negatively can interfere with or grow relatedness and community; therefore, how people experience relating with differences becomes a critical factor in antiracism praxis.

Antiracism is much more than simply not being racist (Kendi 2019). Antiracism includes disrupting centuries-old institutions that perpetuate harm resulting in lifelong and intergenerational racial trauma. Antiracism recognizes and elevates modern and ancestral knowledges and technologies (Farias *et al.* 2020; Leite Junior *et al.* 2021). Importantly, antiracism praxis is not contingent on a single definition of antiracism, antiracism praxis, decolonisation or decolonising occupation. Putting oneself in the antiracist struggle is a political alignment given expression through everyday actions with all people we connect with.

Theorising antiracism: a decolonising occupation, everyday life and action

Despite the well-researched and well-established understandings of race as a social construct and racism as a social determinant that impacts multiple dimensions of life, racism is poorly researched and the impacts on everyday occupation are poorly understood within the profession

(Beagan 2020; Farias *et al.* 2020). Such under-theorisation of racism in relation to occupation, activities, everyday life and ways of life is a predictable outcome of a pro-western-dominated profession (Amorim *et al.* 2020; Costa *et al.* 2020; Farias *et al.* 2020; Johnson & Lavalley 2021; Leite Jr. *et al.* 2021; Martins & Farias 2020; Ramugondo 2018; Ryan *et al.* 2020). While power remains firmly in white knowledge systems, the flip side is that the profession remains under-evolved. Worse still, being miseducated and unengaged with antiracism is causing further racial trauma (e.g. Gordon-Burns & Walker 2015).

Antiracist, decolonial occupational therapies understand that there are many ideas about and practices of occupation, activities, everyday life and ways of life. BIPOC colleagues and allies have contributed to deepening the examination of these diverse concepts (e.g. Amorim *et al.* 2020; Costa 2021; Costa *et al.* 2020; Emery-Whittington 2021; Farias *et al.* 2020; Gibson 2020; Guajardo *et al.* 2015; Leite Jr. *et al.* 2021; Martins 2021; Ramugondo 2018; Ribeiro 2021; Simaan 2020b), and in so doing, they are decolonising the profession's attachment to the need for universal acceptability of a single core understanding of these concepts. Such 'disruptions' to the 'usual' western theorising can both deepen and widen understandings of the potential of occupational therapies.

Certainly, there are no lack of spaces to theorise racism and its impact on occupation, activities, everyday life and ways of life. Yet, due to a lack of positionality and self-critique, the profession tends to overstate the amount and extent of antiracism work done while perpetuating ahistorical, apolitical approaches. Further, if as Bojadžijev (2020: 193) states, institutions maintain and reproduce 'racism as episteme' then we must carefully critique why we are calling on the very same institutions – that maintain and reproduce racism as episteme – to theorise and examine links between racism and occupational therapy core concepts. Indeed, we assert that our profession's particular and special contribution to antiracism work is theorising the links between racism, society, everyday life and occupation.

Lack of theorising seriously challenges the ability of certain parts of the profession to honestly face racism in practice, education and research, but also speaks to the incredible lengths that some colleagues have gone to bring existing theorising to life. For example, Angell (2014: 104) argued for the examination of 'occupation in perpetuating the hegemonic social order', allowing closer attention to the potential of occupation to be a vehicle for the transmission of racism. Ramugondo (2015) expanded thinking further with the contribution of occupational consciousness, grounded in the works of Fanon and Biko. More recently, Ryan *et al.* (2020: 412) argued that '...occupations reflect society, but also...occupations can change society'. Such theorising illuminates and affirms the potential of occupation – once decolonised – as a means to resist colonialism and heal (Emery-Whittington 2021; Gibson 2020; Ryan *et al.* 2020; Simaan 2020b). In addition, Farias *et al.* (2020) reported that social occupational therapy promotes various elaborations for the creation of strategies to strengthen BIPOC individuals and collectives, considering their subjectivities.

To support theorising antiracism within occupational therapy and science we ask: What has been this discipline and profession's contribution to racism? Moreover, what do the racialised tell us? Importantly, when historically excluded communities join with the construction and implementation of antiracism efforts, what do they set as measures of antiracism praxis and why?

In proposing a stepwise programme of collective-centred antiracism that includes antiracism measures, we note that despite the burgeoning literature about antiracism in occupational therapy and occupational science since June 2020, few authors have implemented and evaluated active antiracism in practice. This is important. Antiracism is praxis, and decolonisation is not a metaphor. To borrow from one of the late Audre Lorde's book titles: *The Master's Tools Will Never Dismantle the Master's House*. Therefore, whatever antiracism measures Global North occupational therapy has, they have not dismantled racism and thus a rebuild is required. However, a measure of scepticism is warranted given the gravity and urgency of the task, the overwhelming evidence of racist harms, derailments and delays to date (i.e. focus on cultural competency and diversity), and where much of the hoarded power still very much lies.

Antiracism in five steps: a collectives-centred programme

In a review of effective antiracism approaches, Ben *et al.* (2020) report on the importance of theory-led, evidence-based plans with clear objectives and well-designed evaluation. Coordinated cross-organisation and sector initiatives supported by decision-makers and funders were indicators of successful initiatives. However, the review did not explicate the positionality of the approaches, which means that it is difficult to determine by whose measure the antiracism initiative was successful or not. Crucially, success, achievement and value for BIPOC collectives may not look the same for non-BIPOC persons, and it is no measure of wellbeing to be as 'sick' or as 'well' as non-BIPOC persons.

Step 1: Gather or join with the experts to build your community

Those with the least to gain from racism, and compounded oppression of any kind, are essential to every discussion of antiracism. Active collectives pursuing equity and the end of racism already have the experience, skills, analysis and capacity to support new antiracism initiatives. The unfortunate practice of cherry-picking and collecting BIPOC 'champions' is replaced with a practice of engaging with collectives of champions. For example, in Aotearoa New Zealand, the Teaching Council has partnered with several agencies, including the NZ Human Rights Commission (includes the Race Relations Commission), the Commission for Children, Te Papa National Museum, and other collectives, as powerful partners for its antiracism programme Unteach Racism.

Representation is a vital part of any venture to end racism because, as Came (2014) argues, majoritarian decision-making is a site of racism, often appearing in the guise of democracy as 'numerical fairness'. Conversely, Came (2014) noted that governance discussions involving numerically minoritised groups – often the experts in the room – tend to benefit dominant groups. Listing antiracism agenda items last or delaying 'until the next meeting' has caused numerically minoritised people to report feeling unsafe (Came *et al.* 2019). Numerical fairness arguments mean that hoarded power remains with those that gain from maintaining the racist status quo. Shifting focus to instead highlight why there is an over-representation of those that consciously or unconsciously maintain the status quo is useful (Came *et al.* 2019). We argue for intentional over-representation of BIPOC collectives at every level of decision-making – at every meeting.

A flawed consultation process is a common refrain of historically excluded groups (Came 2014). Instead, collectives resourced to drive the antiracism initiative will ensure BIPOC voices remain centred. In addition, white-washing and erasure of expertise provided are unlikely if decision-making processes (e.g. voting, consensus), framing of issues (e.g.

epistemologies included or not) and evidence collected (e.g. positionality of literature) are carefully considered and agreed on (Came 2014).

The work to end racism is a serious undertaking, so it is expected that everyone involved in the work is politically astute and has a firm understanding of the shape of their contribution, such as skills, experience, time or access to resources. Therefore, it is recommended that allies and BIPOC champions are acknowledged and supported in their own growth, with regular coaching and mentoring and plenty of opportunities to build capacity. For example, a local collective of allies in Aotearoa New Zealand meets monthly to crowdsource solutions to dilemmas or difficulties. The process is a deliberately collective, open, non-blaming space with generous sharing of accumulated wisdom as the norm. Such communities of learning are integral to keeping momentum up, preventing burnout and isolation, and helping to ride through tough times. Came noted in her research that unacknowledged deficiencies in political competency could be a site of racism (Came 2014). Therefore, regular, reliable opportunities for growth ultimately support transparency and accountability across the community.

Effective antiracism plans require ring-fenced, multiply sourced, protected funding for years. Guaranteed long-term funding means that lasting changes based on well-developed plans can be implemented, evaluated, disseminated and improved. Moreover, when the budget is matched with executive and senior level power, then critical institutional decisions and changes occur at what seems lightning speed. Antiracism programmes and collectives must be confidently and continuously supported, with commitment from all levels, but especially senior levels. Antiracism measures may include tracking funding for these initiatives over time, quantifying the decision-making ability, and calculating that the time allotted for these roles is sufficient for antiracism-only initiatives.

Step 2: Collective mapping of racism

To end racism, one has to know where it is and by what means it continues to be reproduced in the space of concern. Occupational therapy emerged and is reproduced from the same societal structures that have racism firmly positioned as the status quo. The hegemonic history of occupational therapy is acknowledged and must not prevent or frame the creation of new ways of acting. That being the case, the honest desire to identify sites of racism, label those sites accordingly, and map those sites in relation to each other, must be bold, sustained and collective.

This means proactive broadening of scope to identify sites of racism and other forms of oppression, varied expressions of racism, and resources that seek to measure and end racism. It is vital that non-English language written and spoken resources, within and outside the profession, are actively sought and engaged with. Although it is uncommon to find instruments that measure and report on the existence of racism inside western-dominated occupational therapy spheres, it does not follow that they do not exist. Examining whose voices are absent and whose are present, how and why that came to be is part of identifying sites of racism.

Mapping sites of racism may be as straightforward as providing safe opportunities for those most affected by racism to report on the sites they are aware of and experienced with. It is our experience that when provided with safe opportunities to map sites of racism, people are able to do so efficiently and without hesitation. As with every space in this work, safety is essential. Further time will be required for in-depth analysis and mapping of the more hidden forms of racism, such as lack of salary or promotion opportunities. More than that, once started, this is a process that is best seen as a series of beginnings: actions sparking actions. Identification and reporting on sites of racism need to be believed, acknowledged, filtered only by those entrusted to do so, and most importantly, prioritised for action where and when required. Mapping sites of racism is potentially a risk to reputation, position, career and personal safety.

Institutional racism is also wielded by silence and the withholding of information, material resources and opportunity (Wingfield & Alston 2014; Blessett & Littleton 2017). Oppression is like a hidden algorithm written skillfully into societal structures. Therefore, open questions like 'In what ways do BIPOC communities thrive here?' may elicit stories of antiracism, resistance to racism and resistance to antiracism. In addition, examination of the effectiveness of current antiracism approaches gives further insight as to the shape and peculiarities of racism of the organisation in question.

Examination of institutional racism would include policies, procedures, curriculum and demographic information of all persons involved or benefitting from the organisation: current students, employees, service users, stakeholders, shareholders, investors and contractors. Available and accurate demographic information means that monitoring at a basic level for diversity policies, quotas and outcomes can occur. However, it is common for such information to be subject to gatekeeping and poorly recorded, again a possible site of racism. In addition, anonymity in feedback through a third party may ensure that truthful feedback is protected from coercion or fear of acts of reprisal, such as losing jobs, poor grades, missing opportunities like promotions, being prematurely discharged from treatment, or not offered all treatment options. Respectful and careful handling of data and information is central to accurate identification of sites of racism.

Step 3: Analyse the stories and numbers

Methods for analysis of data need to be researched, developed and agreed on, allowing room for localisation and change where and when needed. No one single method of analysis is possible or indeed necessary. Importantly, each instance, story and experience shared about sites of racism deserves to be seen as the gift that it is: trauma shared generously in the hope of transformation. Therefore, the analysis and building of antiracism measures call for several safe pairs of hands to hold the space for better. Initiating systemic change can be clarified by knowing exactly where racism resides and being open to addressing change in multiple spheres and interactions alongside an accountable, committed community.

Step 4: Have a plan (or join with those who have a plan)

The planning process can be itself a potential site of healing. Planning to end racism demands the creation of methods that can accurately and sensitively guide antiracism approaches for the given context. Centring BIPOC wellbeing and humanity engages BIPOC imaginations, creativity, generosity and experience. 'The plan' becomes a collection of sequenced moments of co-creation whereby connections are made and renewed, and community is forged.

As a gold standard, we would argue that well-managed, inclusive processes of antiracism initiatives are crucial. The energy, the soul if you like, of these processes, is not tied to neoliberal ideology of ownership and is instead powered by the energy of collectives working and sharing together for the benefit of all. This necessarily requires a different set of tools from those The Master has. The transformational potential required for new tools can already be found in breakthrough collectives. Examples of several of these collectives within occupational therapy are listed in Table 7.1.

Table 7.1: Affinity and collective groups

AbleOTUK	Inspired by BAMEOTUK, AbleOTUK is a UK occupational therapy network/advocacy group for practitioners, students, researchers, educators and people with disabilities/long-term health conditions. Twitter: https://twitter.com/AbleOTUK Website: https://affinot.co.uk/ableotuk
Antiracist OT Collective	Founded by a Métis woman in Canada for the global occupational therapy community, the Antiracist OT Collective is an approach to continuing education that supports participants to engage and reflect on issues that are often complicated and emotional. This approach builds on community support, becoming more self-aware, and socially just occupational therapy professionals. Contact: Angie Phenix: phenixotconsulting@gmail.com
BAMEOTUK	Black, Asian and minoritised occupational therapy staff, students and educators network based in the UK. Twitter: https://twitter.com/BAMEOTUK Podcasts: www.youtube.com/channel/UCKObQkHUl0lCiXgrvn7lg_A
DisruptOT	Founded by a Bengali American woman to disrupt the status quo in occupational therapy by highlighting the work of the global majority in issues of antiracism, decolonisation, gender, sexuality, mental health and community building. The DisruptOT community is open to all with the intention of making critical knowledge free and accessible. Twitter: https://twitter.com/DisruptOT Website: www.disruptot.org
Grupo Dona Ivone Lara: Occupational Therapy and Black Population	Grupo Dona Ivone Lara was created by young occupational therapists who yearned to reflect and produce knowledge about occupational therapy focused on understanding the specificities and the contributions of the profession from the Black community. Instagram: @grdonaivonelara Twitter: @grdonaivonelara

Indigenous OT Consortium	The IOTC is a growing network of indigenous occupational therapists, who have been meeting since 2018, co-convened in unity by First Australians (Chontel Gibson and Corrinne Butler) and Māori (Isla Emery-Whittington and Georgina Davis) colleagues. Contact: Isla Emery-Whittington: isla@whittington.nz
LGBTQIA+OT UK	LGBTQIA+OT UK is a UK-based affinity group, formed by a small group of LGBTQIA+ occupational therapists and occupational therapy students. The network was created as a space to connect, share, learn and celebrate, both for those who identify as LGBTQIA+ as well as for our much-needed allies. Twitter: https://twitter.com/LGBTQIAOTUK Website: https://affinot.co.uk/lgbtqiaotuk
Lab-Iṣẹ́ – African Studies Laboratory	Lab-Iṣẹ́ – African Studies Laboratory aims to bring together different researchers and organisations interested in African epistemologies and activities, seeking to reconstruct Afro-references in occupational therapy that deal with the production of Afro-Brazilian subjectivities. Instagram: @laboratorioise Website: https://iselaboratorio.wixsite.com/laboratorioise
Māori OT Network	The Māori OT Network meets monthly and is primarily about supporting and developing Māori occupational therapy professionals. It centres Māori aspirations and ways of being together and respects tribal difference. It aims to hold annual national events. Contact: Isla Emery-Whittington: isla@whittington.nz
Multicultural, Diversity, and Inclusion Network	The Multicultural, Diversity, and Inclusion Network is a network of independent groups of various diverse identities and affiliations based on race/ethnicity, disability, sexual orientation and religious affiliation which collectively support the increase of diversity and inclusion in occupational therapy within the United States. Website: www.aota.org/practice/manage/multicultural.aspx

cont.

Occupational Therapy and Indigenous Health Network	The Occupational Therapy and Indigenous Health Network (OTIHN) started in 2009 as a volunteer group working with the Canadian Association of Occupational Therapists national office staff to develop supports, resources and lobby efforts to build and promote occupational therapy services with indigenous peoples. Their purpose is to provide leadership, networking and support for occupational therapists collaborating with indigenous clients and communities across Canada. Website: www.caot.ca/site/pd/otn/otahn

Planning to measure antiracism

Like methods to identify sites of identified racism, antiracism measures need to be local and context-specific because racism looks different in different spaces. It is important to be vigilant and avoid falling back into coloniality (Ramugondo 2018) and this will likely require being led by new people and processes. In addition, it makes sense to remain cognizant of – but not necessarily led by – tools and measures of antiracism praxis that already exist.

There is a vast proliferation of tools to support the measurement of antiracism practices available. Importantly, tools have their own genealogy of thought, epistemologies that birth them, frameworks, values and ethics that shape them. Tools selected to guide and support BIPOC collectives to measure antiracism must unapologetically centre BIPOC needs and wants. Many current measures are centred on an individual and their beliefs (e.g. Implicit Association Test), or they rely on accurate recording of ethnic data, salaries and job opportunities. We argue that such measures still primarily only attend to revealing the depth, shape and extent of racial wounds and harms. Antiracism measures built on localised contextual knowledge, data and stories are likely to have several characteristics, including: embedding rights focus, taking for granted that BIPOC communities already employ many methods of resisting racism, consciously building communities of learning, and processes promoting healing through a vast system of collective knowledges and centuries of adept navigation of colonial structures. In addition, an antiracism initiative may include:

- a commitment to being collectives led

- a commitment to engaging all stakeholders

- a commitment to changing structures

- a commitment to promoting accountability and transparency

- a commitment to resource and funding

- a commitment to building public policies that favour historically excluded populations.

Antiracism plans ought to mitigate backlash (Ben *et al.* 2020) against BIPOC collectives and antiracism workers. Regular assessment of agile safeguards that protect staff from racial discrimination, harassment and retaliation from peers, supervisors and service users is central to the plan. In addition, safe reporting of harmful events and their aftermath must capture details of exactly how people reporting harm are protected from reprisal and further injury. The system for tracking racist occurrences will bring visibility to who is being targeted, where and when incidents occur, and prevention strategies, if any. Supports for healing from racialised harm that centre the wellness of racialised services users, students and practitioners would include evidenced processes and detailed data about those that cause racial harm (accidentally or otherwise).

Antiracism plans are transparent, available and updated regularly. Complete transparency at all levels means that racism cannot seep in and hide. Having then gathered the antiracism community, identified and mapped the sites of racism (which includes bespoke methods of analysis of the sites of racism), and co-created a plan (that centres BIPOC aspirations and has carefully selected antiracism measures of success), it is time to mobilise the plan.

Step 5: Action, reflection, action
The next action is the best action. In other words, do something regularly, evaluate that action, adjust when needed, plan the next action, and repeat. Getting and staying stuck, accepting delay and waiting for 'staff development and training' have been effective in maintaining racist structures and processes. What is clear is that most Global North bastions of occupation studies have yet to show significant impact as a result of sustained antiracism programmes and initiatives. However, there are a number of antiracism initiatives and projects that occupational therapy professionals are engaged in and lead in the Global

South and in spaces unchained to Global North spaces. It is possible that antiracism actions are being effectively and consciously positioned for maximum effect.

We argue that there is an urgent need for humble representation and role-modelling of antiracism as central to development of accountability across the profession. The construction of legitimacy in the profession is often formed around individual activities such as conferences and congresses (Guajardo *et al.* 2015). It is important that antiracism initiatives and measures are not captured and pigeonholed by that kind of colonising process. Instead, we encourage collectives and allies as role models to take care with selecting where and why they present and share, by what means their work is given a platform, and what the risks and gains are of sharing.

Greater diversity and representation in health practitioners will result in better care for service users and offer a more well-rounded education for future practitioners, particularly increasing the likelihood of success for BIPOC students (Milner 2006; Ridgeway & McGee 2018). This begs the question as to why there are not more BIPOC students accepted into occupational therapy programmes as reflected in society. Carefully curated occupational therapy courses that are co-designed to be experienced as antiracist, anti-ableist and LGBTQIA+ friendly are possible spaces to influence profession-level change. It is still to be seen if it is a worthwhile endeavour to take existing courses and build/add in such societal and cultural change.

Though it is not yet well documented in occupational therapy research, other services have shown that culture matching results in better care. Matching service users to mental health providers with similar racial and ethnic backgrounds has resulted in better outcomes, satisfaction and service utilisation (Meyer & Zane 2013). Hence, monitoring for fair representation in local, national and international spaces is an important aspect of antiracism actions. Unfortunately, when faced with opportunities to increase diversity, it is noted that the profession tends to favour colleagues from mainstream Global North ahead of Global South. Representation alone is not a measure of antiracism. We also assert that cultural competency efforts are not antiracism strategies in that knowledge of culture in practice does not by itself mitigate the impacts of racism (Allen 2010).

The time to act is now. There have been many lessons from this pandemic moment in history. Besides the glaring inequities in income and job protection, border rules and medical resources, vaccine availability has highlighted global inequities. Vaccine inequity has shown 'you can't put out half a fire', and it is the same for racism and oppression; a plan to end some but not all oppression is no plan at all. No one is safe from a fire until everyone is.

Conclusion

We recognise the expertise and multi-dimensional range of BIPOC collectives within the profession that have already begun to mobilise and disrupt racism. Antiracist and disruptive action in the current world puts us in dialogue with the constant contradiction and tension in institutions and with those who propagate racism on an everyday basis. Therefore, the proposal of an antiracist action and the possibility of measuring actions comes in a movement of conscientisation, sum of forces and composition of a struggle that is bigger and needs many bodies to face it.

If the reader requires, there is a plethora of workplace, practice and research tools that can support the identification and measurement of 'bias,' opportunity, trauma and consequence of racism (or not). However, we would caution against a reach for antiracism measures ahead of:

- mobilising the expertise of antiracism collectives, with high-level backing

- attaining a full and comprehensive cultural understanding of the organisation and its particular expressions of racism through mapping

- planning effective antiracism actions and evaluation of those actions

- taking sound actions that not only align but are led by BIPOC aspirations.

This antiracism approach and suggestions for antiracism measures are posed *by* BIPOC colleagues *to* BIPOC colleagues *for* BIPOC colleagues and proven allies. We encourage colleagues to complicate thinking, strategise thoroughly, mobilise multiple collectives as one, and be invested for the long haul as we reconstruct the profession to theorise racism and honestly meet injustices. This chapter seeks to broaden and contribute to antiracist action in education, professional practice and research in occupational therapy, based on our particular experiences. Thus, it is not about producing a kind of protocol, following a recipe or crossing a finish line in the hope of solving inequities. We can't hold every hand that joins the path of the everyday struggle, but by your actions of disruption we will know you.

Farias *et al.* (2020: 245) asserted:

Part of this is seeing, in the occupational therapist, the duty of social articulator, enabling people to know their rights and understand themselves as capable of carrying out transformational movements. In other words, it is about being a facilitator across art, culture, leisure, health, education, knowledge spaces with strategies to confront racial inequality and racism, thus upholding social rights.

Reflective quadrant: Identifying, recording and understanding learning from the chapter

What? (Describe what have I learnt)

Relevance? (Why is this topic relevant to me/to my practice? Relate/align to/with, e.g., research literature, professional bodies' proficiencies/competencies, service delivery/service user benefit, legislation – briefly and critically discuss)

How will this learning change me/my practice?

What actions do I have to follow up on to develop my learning in this area or apply to my practice? (SMART goal format or similar)

Appendix: Positionality

The invitation to write this chapter presents us with several pleasant challenges. We are three people from different countries, so writing this chapter is a process of approximation, dialogue and mutual learning. One author is a cisgender, gay, Latin American man who lives in Brazil and was able to enter the public university due to the social policies of quotas, access and permanence. The other authors are cisgender, heterosexual women, one a first generation Bengali American and the other Māori, with responsibilities to her tribal community and Māori peer network. We each share a commitment to support the growing BIPOC occupational therapy global communities. Two of the authors experience English as a secondary language. The language also crossed us, with everything involved in it. Although this text arrives to you in English, it was also thought and elaborated on in Brazilian Portuguese and Māori, thus requiring delicate translation of theorising from different languages and ideologies.

The possibility of being able to write about occupational therapy, racism, and its marks in everyday life and in the subjects' occupations, is a privilege, but also a painful process of excavation. This means revisiting current and past racial trauma, theorising, and transforming these into action – into the possibility of change – in order to promote a better world for racialized people. Each of the authors has undeservedly experienced aggression in different dimensions and overt racism while training, practising and/or researching occupational therapy. We have used several strategies over many years to resist, heal and overcome the effects of racism, including founding DisruptOT global collective, Māori OT Network, Dona Ivone Lara Group, and many more.

CHAPTER 8

Active Antiracist Allyship in Occupational Therapy

Ryan Lavalley, Marie-Lyne Grenier, Kirsty Stanley, David Marsden

Introduction

Before we move into our chapter it is important that we state that we acknowledge we are white authors who have been invited to critically discuss antiracism and allyship relatively freely, which is of itself a huge privilege. We must understand that our allyship journey will require an intentional and lifelong process of unlearning, genuine community-building, and willingness to deconstruct power structures that continue the centring of whiteness. The reverberating quote from the late Martin Luther King Jr., American minister and civil rights activist, indicates the responsibility of an ally:

> The ultimate measure of a person is not where one stands in moments of comfort and convenience, but where one stands in times of challenge and controversy. (King 1963: 20)

While we recognize that allyship is not just for white people, we write this chapter from a white perspective, as befits our positionalities. This chapter is an invitation to consider with us how we, as a professional community, can move forward in this important allyship work to disrupt racism, inequity and injustice. A critical antiracist lens calls occupational therapy practitioners to move beyond a neoliberal or 'cultural competency' approach (Grenier 2020; Razack 1995), which is often seen in 'implicit bias' training approaches (Dobbin & Kalev 2018), and step into the realm of advocacy and targeted actions aimed at policy and social change (Kendi 2019).

This chapter is guided by the following two questions:

- What is antiracist allyship and how can it contribute to addressing systemic racism in occupational therapy?

- How can we, as occupational therapists, embody authentic antiracist allyship in our everyday practice?

Meaning of antiracist allyship

Everyone is implicated in reproducing racist harms.

We define antiracist allyship as an ongoing collective process aimed at eliminating racist harms. We invite readers not to conflate being 'antiracist' with a fixed or set identity but rather as disruptive actions against racist structures, policies and norms. As Lamont (2021) states, 'Saying you're an ally is much easier than actually being an ally. Saying you're an ally looks good on paper, especially if you're never questioned about your inaction.' Allyship describes the actions of those who have more power and/or privilege in socio-political/economic contexts to deconstruct and counteract the racist, oppressive and discriminatory status quo created and maintained by that power and privilege. That being said, we should always consider the heterogeneous experiences within these contexts by adopting an intersectional approach in any allyship work (Crenshaw 1989, 2017). Antiracist allyship must move beyond actions at an interpersonal level to include actions that target policies and structures (Kendi 2019). As occupational therapists, naming the structural, political and economic causes of occupational injustices is vital to moving our profession towards antiracist action (Lavalley & Robinson Johnson 2022; Ramugondo 2015; Bailliard 2016; Simó Algado et al. 2016). Antiracist allyship requires coalition-building and organising collectively against inequities, and should be led by those most impacted by oppressive systems. It requires being vulnerable and human, building authentic relationships that are situated in the deep and systematic complexities of the struggle.

In some contexts, the term 'accomplice' or 'accompliceship' is preferred to 'allyship', to emphasize the actions or inactions, at times subversive or risky, that aim to deconstruct systems of racism and oppression alongside those that they oppress (Suyemoto et al. 2020; Vachon & McConnell 2018).

An occupational therapy practice that embodies an authentic antiracist ethical stance

Models of allyship can sometimes be helpful as introductions to antiracism work (Kendi 2019; Tolliver 2020; Coghill 2021; Lamont 2021). However, they can often give a false sense of security and encourage complacency. Such models can focus too deeply on the experiences of white people and their positions of power without demonstrating active and effective ways to transfer or deconstruct that power (Dabiri 2021). Drawing on our collective experiences, we propose five key principles for antiracist allyship work that position the work as a lifelong political and ethical commitment steeped in contextual complexities:

- Root actions in relationships and decolonial ethics.

- Actively seek education.

- Name the problem, frame the cause.

- Hold up the critical mirror.

- Find your place in the work.

These principles are not intended to form a linear practice but rather describe important dynamic interconnected approaches to the practice of antiracist allyship. This work must centre the communities affected by racism, collaborating with them to lead the changes for antiracism and equity, and therefore will look differently in different contexts and spaces. We invite readers to consider whether suggestions included in this chapter are appropriate for their specific context(s).

Root actions in relationships and decolonial ethics

As Ramugondo (2020) says:

> [...] we were unapologetic about the work being Black led, but that was not accepted. It was viewed as divisive. Almost a swear-word. But if we were only just feminists fighting for inclusion, would men be tasked with leading that inclusion? Well, if that is allowed, then we must expect that it would be inclusion, only on men's terms. Black led does not mean white exclusion. It merely means for a change white people need to learn to follow. Is that a crime?

Most allyship models call for the transfer/sharing of power from those in positions of privilege/influence to those whose power has been taken or oppressed. Equally important – yet rarely discussed – is the development of a deep relational and decolonial ethic that attends to power dynamics consistently, especially during processes (Phenix & Grenier 2020). Ndlovu-Gatsheni (2015: 485) refers to decoloniality as a long-standing political and epistemological movement that is aimed at the 'liberation of (ex-) colonized people from global coloniality'. To achieve a decolonial aim, a deconstruction of existing structures and processes must occur and be followed by a rebuilding, both of which must be led by marginalised communities with the support of those with more power (Bell 2018). This perspective challenges us to consistently be vigilant for the ways in which Eurocentric and colonising approaches are being overvalued or prioritised both prior to and during process.

For example, processes and initiatives currently being adopted in many occupational therapy spaces[1] that target antiracism are historically rooted in white supremacy culture and continue to be overwhelmingly led by white individuals. This is the case for many of our occupational therapy practice process frameworks. These are often driven by and rooted in white centric/Eurocentric perspectives (American Occupational Therapy Association 2021, 2020; Hammell 2009; Townsend *et al.* 2007). We cannot expect to achieve antiracist outcomes while using the same processes that have always sustained white supremacy. Changing this entrenched process requires accountability to people, not institutions. Processes need to change if we want outcomes to change and, as Ramugondo (2020) aptly points out, this change requires non-white leadership. As such, relationships and decolonial approaches must be prioritized (i.e. form the basis for change). We must actively, intentionally and respectfully develop real, honest relationships with community members, colleagues, students, classmates and family most affected by racism, while being vigilant about colonising processes. We must declare as white allies, or potential ones, that we see you our Black and minoritised racialised peers and service users and we will act collaboratively instead of leaving the actions of disruption solely to our Black and minoritised racialised colleagues.

---

1   These may include educational, clinical, community, research, governmental or any other spaces where occupational therapy practitioners participate.

Thinking about process as an outcome (Marie-Lyne)

I completed a doctoral course about 'critical race theory in education' that revolutionised the way I thought about antiracist pedagogy. As a result of this new learning, I added the book *White Fragility* by Robin DiAngelo (2018) as mandatory reading for an undergraduate occupational therapy course I was teaching.

Many students (later I realised they were all white) thanked me for my teaching approach and for introducing them to *White Fragility*. I felt good about myself and that I had made a real change, until a conversation with a small group of students from minoritised racial identities on the last day of class. 'Thank you for broaching these topics,' one student said, 'but I have to say, I didn't really learn much from reading the book.' Seeing the look of confusion on my face, they elaborated. 'I live this stuff every day. So, I didn't really learn anything. Maybe you're catering your readings to a white audience? I mean, the author is white, and the book is really meant for a white audience.'

Had I reflected more about my *process*, I would have understood that it was entirely white-led, Eurocentric and accountable to an institution (university), rather than those most affected by racism. As a result, my process created racist, exclusionary and oppressive outcomes for a significant proportion of the students in my class. What would my students' learning experience have been if the course had been Black-led, included readings by Black or authors from minoritised racial identities or was accountable to the people most affected by racism? How would I have had to change my process?

Marie-Lyne's story highlights that the positioning of the serious 'job' of white allies is to decentre and not reinforce whiteness and the privilege and power imbalance that comes with it (Cole 2021), in order to be actively antiracist, anti-discriminatory and anti-oppressive. As allies, we need to be hyper alert to not being performative, tokenistic or narrow in discussions, teachings or actions regarding racism and forms of inequity and injustice, so as not to reinforce white centrism and further marginalise and harm colleagues and students of BME heritage backgrounds.

Actively seek education

Education is not just the consumption of resources but is an ongoing and iterative process. Embrace the value in consistently incorporating deep, critical and open-minded learning in your antiracist allyship journey. Rushing in with uninformed, easy or 'performative' actions is likely to lead to misguided and potentially more harmful white centring outcomes (Noman 2020). Importantly, within the profession, this learning must be modelled and practised by occupational therapy leaders, regulators, educators, practitioners, students and researchers.

Practitioners must actively seek to understand the social, political, historical and economic systems that impact the lives of us all (and continue to do so), especially minoritised and marginalised groups. Be curious and ask questions, such as how are occupations racialised in our society? Questioning is important in our understanding of the root of some occupational injustices (Pollard & Sakellariou 2014). It is important to seek out the perspectives of those who aim to deconstruct and educate about the realities of racism and whiteness and who challenge us to consider and connect to our own racialised experiences.

Although there may be a paucity of literature discussing the effects of structural racism on occupation, some of the available occupation-centred literature can be found in the references of this book. The limited literature makes us think about who is gatekeeping the knowledge and what the topics are that are pushed forward by the lead scholars' writings, because this could also be reinforcing the structural racism and discrimination in the profession. A wealth of resources about racism, antiracism and white supremacy is available for those willing to look beyond our professional writings, or what Turcotte and Holmes (2021) call our own 'disciplinary propaganda'. This includes wider sources (e.g. news, b/vlogs, books and podcasts). Dabiri (2021: 111) also points to the power of fiction in immersing readers in the lives of others, in containing 'profound truths about the human condition', and in exploring the 'interiority' and intersectionality of individual people, while also acting as a 'portal to' other antiracist actions. Diversifying and critically reviewing our social media consumption is also important (Dabiri 2021). We must celebrate and amplify the contributions in art, music, dance, film, science, technology, business and politics of minoritised people and groups. By doing so, we recognise the incredible resilience that communities have been forced to cultivate, as well as the important societal contributions they have made throughout history in all spheres of life.

Education can come from direct interactions with people about their experiences, but we have to balance the line between knowledge extraction and exploitation and getting an education. This requires a nuanced and intentional approach, and we should critically reflect on our responses, especially when we are not expecting to be educated. When confronted about – particularly our own – racism, we can do more harm than good with our reactions. We can experience defensive white guilt/hurt/victimhood/tears, but we must not focus on the minoritised and marginalised groups to help us work through this and burden them further. We must use those feelings to mobilise us into educating ourselves further and engaging in actions aimed at antiracism which in turn will reduce these feelings (Accapadi 2007). Oluo (2017) challenges white people in particular to be more open, receptive and responsive to feedback and critique.

There may be times when we would like to seek education from an individual or group directly to help us in our allyship efforts. Here are some considerations:

- Before asking questions of a minoritised person or group, first seek education from materials that already exist.

- Pause and check in on why you are searching for the answer. Are your questions based on racist presumptions? Is finding the answer more about making you feel better?

- Remember that through relationships, shared occupations and community building, an answer to your question may organically emerge.

- Consider who to ask. Is there a trusted person who will hold you accountable and help unpack your question? Are you in a situation or space where it is appropriate to ask for this education?

- Seek permission to ask. Take no offence if someone does not want to offer education or to answer. It is not their responsibility or obligation.

- Actively listen and learn, rather than debate or justify. Hear the experience, then reflect. There is no place for the 'devil's advocate' here.

There is a time and place to unpack our own experiences and mistakes, sometimes with others who are practising allyship and sometimes with those who are from minoritised groups. Patience, intentionality and a willingness to be uncomfortable are necessary but we have to also move into antiracist actions/activities.

Evaluating our reading/education (Kirsty)

My immediate response to the novel *The Hate U Give* (Thomas 2017) was that it needed to have a more *balanced* narrative. The book is told solely from a Black teen girl's perspective after seeing a friend get shot by police. On reflection, I see how my privilege came into play with this reaction. It didn't matter if the white cop was a 'bad guy' or someone who made a split-second decision, or even that we heard his point of view; this book was rightly focused on the experience and voice of the Black characters. The fact is, the main character's story could not be told without acknowledging her experience of racism and its impact on her life.

As a profession that prides itself on being person-centred, we must centre the narratives of minoritised individuals and groups (including colleagues), understand how racism affects their experience, how our actions or inactions within systems contribute, and change our practices accordingly.

Kirsty's narrative started with centring whiteness, decentring and reducing the seriousness of the main issue of the institutional racism in the police system emboldening the police officer to shoot and kill a Black male teen. This was instead of centring the very racist topic of demonising Black youths as criminals because they are Black, which sometimes leads to fatal consequences for the unarmed Black males (Smiley & Fakunle 2016). Kirsty reflected and recentred the main issue of institutional racism within the story and expanded this to the further needs of the profession to deal with racism.

Placing a critical whiteness studies lens on both Marie Lyne's and Kirsty's stories helps to examine how the structures and cultures that privilege white people can be analysed as a source of systemic racism and oppression (Matias & Boucher 2021). One viewpoint is that this type of examination is not recentring whiteness, nor excluding Black people and scholars. For example, some Black scholars such as Fanon, Mills and Dumas instruct that critical whiteness is centring Black humanity as action to disrupt racism, inequity and injustice (Matias & Boucher 2021).

Name the problem, frame the cause

Where we have often stumbled in antiracism allyship is in appropriately framing racism as the problem rather than race. Historic and ongoing disparities experienced by minoritised people exist in virtually every system in our societies; in employment rates (Bertrand & Mullainathan 2004), discipline in schools (Edwards 2016), incarceration (Alexander 2010), autism diagnoses (Burkett *et al.* 2015), and even the make-up of the occupational therapy profession (American Occupational Therapy Association 2014). These are consequences of institutional racism. The permeating lie of racism is that race inherently causes particular differences or outcomes.

No outcomes should be predictable based on race because race is not a biologically based characteristic and is only constructed via racism (Lang 2000). White people are particularly implicated in the perpetuation of these fallacies, especially when we lack the relational and decolonial ethics and structural understandings described earlier. In North America, we see the construction of race and racism tied deeply to religious identities, proselytization (religious indoctrination), the rise of capitalism, and the trans-Atlantic trade of enslaved peoples (Cannon 2008). In the UK, we have seen racism constructed with classism, ethnic groups and national identities (Allen 2012; Beagan & Chacala 2012). Currently in Ontario (Canada), indigenous children are 2.6 times more likely to be placed in foster care than their population proportion; Black children 2.2 times higher (Ontario Human Rights Commission 2018). Race was and is used to justify dehumanising, kidnapping and enslaving African peoples, and in the subjugation and genocide of indigenous peoples. However, race did not exist before racism (Lang 2000). Racism offers race as a quick, incorrect and dehumanising answer to the question of 'Why is it that certain groups of people have vastly different experiences and outcomes in our world?' (Bell 1993).

At times, seemingly innocuous 'everyday actions' (Lavalley & Robinson Johnson 2022; Ramugondo 2015) within our profession that name the problem but fail to frame the cause can reinforce racist ideas, leading to very real harms. Therefore, acknowledging the problem is so important, but appropriately framing the cause is crucial, and actions to embed antiracism fundamental. For example, while still acknowledging disparities, we could perpetuate fallacies that assume certain groups in the BME populations are worse parents. If we remove race as an option to explain these differences, we are forced to ask harder questions, contextualise systems and historicise the realities in which we live, and we are left with the question: now we know what we know, what are we going to do about it (Kendi 2017, 2019)?

Racist explanations (Ryan)

In the United States, a common racist stereotype is that Black fathers are not present in Black families (Coles & Green 2010; Smith 2017). When I was an occupational therapy fieldwork student, I had just finished working with a young Black teenager accompanied by his mother. In the staff office, a nurse commented, 'We see so many fathers who aren't there for families like them. It really is a shame.' As a 'well-meaning ally', I began offering explanations for this disparity, such as disproportionate arrest rates and imprisonment, employment discrimination, even so far as recounting the removal of men from Black families since the time of enslavement.

I offered reason after reason that justified, yet confirmed, the perception that Black fathers were largely absent from their families. All of these factors and oppressive mechanisms were and are true; however, my explanation still functioned on the assumption that Black fathers are not present in Black families, when, in fact, this stereotype is not true (Coles & Green 2010; Jones & Mosher 2013; Smith 2017) and most Black fathers in the United States are present in their families and in actuality are more engaged in the care of their children than all other racialised groups (Jones & Mosher 2013).

If I had actively sought education to understand the dispari-ty's cause, rather than simply believing the one offered, I would have discovered that the disparity did not even exist. Racism told me that Black families were always worse off and this stereotype had to be true. While Black Americans still face many disparities and unequal outcomes, this was not one of them.

Overstepping my place: learning from mistakes

Another time, I was working with a group of classmates writing a discussion board post about antiracism work in occupational therapy. There was disagreement about the wording and about how direct or 'harsh' we should be in naming and framing our position on the issues discussed versus offering more cushioning around our points to make them more palatable to our classmates.

Unfortunately, when I tried to 'listen to' and amplify the voices of two classmates from minoritised groups, the discussion turned into a debate between white classmates. On reflection, I realised I had stepped out of place by *speaking for*, rather than *holding space* for them to discuss and lead with their perspec-tives. I went back to apologise for taking up so much space in the conversation and committed to working harder to be supportive without overstepping in future.

Listening, paying attention to how my classmates were react-ing, and considering that support did not look like taking over the conversation would have changed the dynamic entirely.

Thinking about Ryan's story through the lens of critical whiteness, the reaction could be related to white saviourism. White saviourism is a modernist notion of altruism based on the universal notion of compas-sion and being selfless (Burr 2010), and as Yu (2021) states, white saviour-ism is actions by the privileged with the aim to centre the minoritised. However, Willer-Kherbaoui (2019) says that through white saviourism, institutional racism gets recycled, because it centres whiteness, and marginalises further, decentring the minoritised people by assuming they do not have agency or power. Ryan took a pause and stopped the false narrative by unlearning racism and learning antiracism as a praxis of resistance and solidarity.

Hold up the critical mirror

We have already stated that 'everyone is racist'. When we say this, we do not imply that everyone overtly and intentionally practises behaviours that oppress people from minoritised groups but rather that we are all actively participating in racist systems. Racism adapts and shifts in order to apply consistent support to racist structures and norms. Therefore, practising antiracist allyship requires us to consistently and critically attend to the potential form shifter that racism can be, including within our own profession. Lifting a mirror to honestly evaluate our ideas and beliefs can be unsettling and requires challenging long-held habits and assumptions (Oluo 2017). This re-evaluation is more than taking an implicit bias test or training at your workplace (Hagiwara *et al.* 2020); we must historicise racism both within and outside the profession and tie those histories to the current socio-political and economic contexts in which we live, work and play (Kendi 2019; Lavalley & Robinson Johnson 2022).

As we adopt a critical lens, we should expect to feel uncomfortable. Acknowledging and appropriately managing this discomfort in a way that fosters growth is key. Reactions based in *White Fragility* (DiAngelo 2018) – a series of defensive mechanisms frequently used by white people to distract from or minimise our racist words and actions, including overly emotional or shocked reactions, centring our own experiences ('I have also faced...') (Lamont 2021), and disregarding individual experiences (Coghill 2021) – should be avoided. Developing readiness to receive feedback and respond with gratitude, rather than defensiveness, is key (Lamont 2021; Oluo 2017). These genuine and honest conversations are valuable tools in coalition building and creating supportive, reparative relationships. Resmaa Menakem (n.d.) describes that no matter what our skin colour, we should practise somatic abolitionism. Resmaa describes this as an ancestral return to 'human bodies respecting, honoring, and resonating with other human bodies' for relational culture building through united antiracist practices and processes, to disrupt the structural and interpersonal harms on minoritised bodies due to racism oppression and injustices (Menakem n.d., 2022). That is, using our bodies as collective collaborative vessels to resist (Menakem 2022). Resmaa continues that any white body can be a living embodiment of antiracism, of white body somatic abolitionism, through considered and persistent repetition of actions, sometimes failing, sometimes being successful, but always moving forward; it is the collective collaborative connections that keep you going (Menakem 2022). From a further critical perspective, we can more effectively analyse our actions, as well as those of others, across interrelated dimensions of society at the micro, meso and macro levels.

Macro: Our profession's people and knowledge

The ethnic diversity within the profession globally – and particularly in predominantly white countries, is not representative of our populations, or indeed always measured (American Occupational Therapy Association 2014; NHS Digital 2022). This is especially true of those in leadership positions of professional organisations. Furthermore, globally, Eurocentric knowledge rooted in predominantly white experiences is often presented as dominant or foundational in occupational therapy (Fijal & Beagan 2019; Guajardo Córdoba 2020). For example, make a racial heat map of authors to start to re-address balance between knowledges of the Global South and North footprint within the occupational therapy curriculum. Active allyship, and a critical perspective, require that we ask and find answers to why we allow the status quo to exist, and then go on to effectively disrupt it. This involves collecting data and informing antiracist work with that data. Leadership and authority within the profession require more equitable redistribution, beyond proportional representation based on population. Actively addressing oppressive dynamics that impact both served populations and colleagues requires being led by and amplifying power for practitioners who have been and continue to be oppressed and excluded.

Meso: Recruitment and selection processes

Issues of equity and diversity within occupational therapy workplaces are important to consider. These include, but are not limited to, the hiring and selection process (Catlin 2021), which is broadly white-centric in western countries (Guajardo Córdoba 2020; Hammell 2009), racist through a variety of mechanisms (Bertrand & Mullainathan 2004; Sensoy & DiAngelo 2017), and does not often manage interviewer biases or implicit racist assumptions, policies and practices. Examining processes that we have considered 'fair' through a critically antiracist lens can help reveal the ways in which certain processes and expectations disadvantage those who are not white and potentially how those same processes were rooted in a surreptitious attempt to exclude individuals or groups from minoritised ethnicities from professional roles. These same critiques ought to be considered in regard to admission processes in occupational therapy education. For example, ask domain experts from minoritised heritage to criticise your application, recruitment and selection processes and paperwork, to identify exclusionary and discriminatory language perpetuating institutional racism.

Micro: Critically analysing individual biases

We work in teams and with service users from diverse groups. Norms and routines we take for granted (e.g. eating with a knife and fork), or may not consider (e.g. donning a hijab), often actively exclude, disadvantage or oppress others (Beagan & Etowa 2009). We must critically examine these to support effective antiracist advocacy and relationships. Practising allyship, if someone from a minoritised ethnicity is being targeted or harmed by someone's words or actions in front of you, often means deploying bystander interventions that de-escalate and protect the person being targeted first (Sue *et al.* 2019) and then being an upstander (recognising injustices and using your own capacity to make it right (Johnson *et al.* 2021)) by addressing the wrongdoer if warranted and/or requested. Pulling someone aside or having a personal conversation later to talk through the issue can be helpful. Sharing what you have learned during your allyship work can help support and inform the person who made the mistake. For example, in a team meeting you might raise your own learning on structural racism and ask others if they can see any problems with current structures or processes. While we will not unpack situational strategies here, many resources offer further education on these de-escalation strategies within allyship (American Friends Service Committee 2021; Ihollaback 2021; Sue *et al.* 2019).

Holding up the critical mirror (David)

A member of my team who is Muslim and from a minoritised background was struggling to find a quiet space to pray during Ramadan. They didn't ask for help, but I didn't think to offer help. Viewing this through my lens of an agnostic in a self-proclaimed Christian country, I did not fully recognise the importance of

> this occupation to this person, or the extra challenges they faced institutionally regarding their Muslim identity.
>
> I would now seek to take antiracist actions in our workspace; to use my white privilege to challenge organisational barriers and support my colleagues to find a place to pray.

Just as in critical race theory, in critical whiteness studies, stories enable us to reflect, review and analyse to understand where racism has occurred, how it has been enabled and plan a way forward for structural and institutional change to disrupt racism (Cole 2021).

Find your place in the work

Antiracist allyship requires decentring whiteness and pausing prior to and in the midst of action to evaluate who is going to benefit (Kendi 2019). Would you consider not applying for a position, in which you knew historically BIPOC candidates were never successful, if you knew BIPOC candidates were applying? Would you consider for any sort of interviews sharing the interview questions with all the candidates in advance of the interview? Pausing can be a powerful tool to both deconstruct our own motivations, as well as prevent the continuation of oppressive cycles and systems of white supremacy. Consider the strategy of white caucuses (Roots of Justice 2014); these could take the form of meetings with other white occupational therapists in order to examine issues of whiteness (e.g. white privilege, white saviour complex), hold each other accountable, and identify group and individual strategies for antiracist allyship. These meetings aim to remove the burdens of education and our emotional struggles with antiracist allyship work from our minoritised peers.

Being white does not mean we have not struggled or have struggles or we cannot know anything about racism. We are just as immersed in racism as everyone else; it is about positioning ourselves in, and deconstructing racism from, our privileged angle. Antiracism allyship requires constant and conscious questioning of our own position in the work. Within occupational therapy practice, this requires an acknowledgement that our profession is rooted in white supremacy, that it can and does cause real harm, and that our current 'professional pillars' (models, practice frameworks, assessments, etc.) require reviewing, reframing and rebuilding from an antiracist lens (Grenier 2020).

Importantly, we must reflect on our sphere of influence and where we can best contribute to realistic and effective change. Racism is a complex and nuanced problem that will not be solved within our lifetime or with simple, individualistic solutions. Real change happens over generations. Our individual antiracist actions are small contributions to larger movements and can often be integrated into everyday life (Frank & Muriithi 2015; Ryan *et al.* 2020; Simaan 2017). Determine the most sustainable and effective approach and focus your energy there.

Burgess (1996) warns us of the *myth of progress* in relation to antiracism/anti-oppressive work. There is no one right answer in how to do this work; some situations require us to step back, support and hold space, while others require action, amplification and active accountability. Deep, active and consistent listening with a willingness to be led is essential for effective antiracist allyship. However, being led by the experiences and voices of those oppressed by racism does not mean they should have to hold our hand through the whole process; we are also immersed in racist structures and can learn to critically examine them and act accordingly.

Conclusion: Failing forward

Antiracism in practice requires a healthy dose of scepticism regarding the concept of progress. Burgess (1996) challenges our popular view of progress as linear and always leaning towards improvements in outcomes. Indeed, racism is insidious, often shifting forms in subtle ways and requiring complex interrogation, with relatively unchanged harmful effects. We will often be tripped up in achieving 'progress' by unseen or surreptitious racist structures and systems. We will make mistakes; we are only human. Intersectional groups forming allyship coalitions can better seek to dismantle the structural racism, sexism, ableism and heterosexism that excludes individuals and thwarts equity. Allyship requires us to learn from them, and see beyond our dominant narratives of progress, to better uncover and attend to the increasingly insidious ways that racism and oppression operate in our modern world.

We must understand that we have 'failed forward' (and likely will continue to do so) in many ways in our antiracism work; however, it is important in ensuring that we learn from our mistakes, prevent future ones, and continuously grow with our communities.

Reflective quadrant: Identifying, recording and understanding learning from the chapter

What? (Describe what have I learnt)	**Relevance?** (Why is this topic relevant to me/to my practice? Relate/align to/with, e.g., research literature, professional bodies' proficiencies/competencies, service delivery/service user benefit, legislation – briefly and critically discuss)
How will this learning change me/my practice?	**What actions do I have to follow up on to develop my learning in this area or apply to my practice?** (SMART goal format or similar)

CHAPTER 9

Going Forwards

Magno Nunes Farias and Odeth Richardson

Introduction

Amen Izekor (2020) in her blog post entitled 'Oops, there goes that corporate knee' conjures up images of the death of a career, the death of hopes and aspirations in institutions where racism is rife. She admonishes the managers and boards who often found ways of shying away from calling out blatant racism within their organisations. Occupational therapists must not be rubber-necking bystanders watching the injustices happening to BAME populations they are supposed to work with. The occupational therapy community needs to collaborate, locally, regionally, nationally and globally to do the hard labour of antiracism impactfully. As Nelson Mandela, former President of South Africa, political leader and activist, stated, we are all responsible to each other for each other's ability to exist justly in society:

> For to be free is not merely to cast off one's chains,
> but to live in a way that respects and enhances the freedom of others.
> (2011: 158)

This chapter aims to provoke occupational therapists about the challenges and possibilities of conducting antiracist practice. Many people, including occupational therapists, claim to be non-racist, a noncommittal position. However, the challenge in a racialised society is to be antiracist – in addition to not reproducing racism, it is necessary to develop collaborative collectives as active agents to create a momentum for impactful change globally which every day go against racism. The motivational words of Michelle Obama, former first lady of the United States, ring true here, as we need courage to move forward and hope to re-imagine a better world, an actively antiracist occupational therapy profession:

> History has shown us that courage can be contagious,
> and hope can take on a life of its own. (2011)

The challenge is not simple and requires theoretical and methodological strategies from professionals to operationalize antiracist practices (Farias *et al.* 2018; Farias & Lopes 2020; Lavalley & Robinson Johnson 2022).

Thus, the questions that guide this chapter are:

- How do we sustain antiracism in occupational therapy?

- Why must occupational therapy professionals show they are committed to antiracist practice?

- How does the profession demonstrate and engage in antiracist strategising systemically?

To answer these questions, examples of two realities of occupational therapy will be given from the UK and Brazil.

Issues of the UK

In the UK, Black History Month is celebrated in October and often the month is used to highlight events and issues affecting the public and workers from BAME populations. These issues then appear forgotten/go under the radar for the next 11 months, until October the following year. Racism is with us every day of the year and it is imperative that actions to address these issues are embedded in our societal and organisational cultures. These issues need to be addressed continuously. Occupational therapy, as a profession within the UK, is largely seen as white, female and middle class dominated. It has been a long journey to get us to this point of challenging the status quo and inaction in occupational therapy. But recent events, Black Lives Matter (BLM) and the COVID-19 pandemic, have brought this situation to the fore again and racism is now being talked about by the profession (e.g. Farias *et al.* 2018; Grenier 2020; Sterman & Njelesani 2021).

The occupational therapy profession has always championed inclusivity through person-centredness, working to enable people to thrive in their lives. It is disappointing that in the code of ethics of the Royal College of Occupational Therapists (RCOT) (2021b), antiracism and social justice are not explicitly identified, just the usual terms equality and diversity. The standards of proficiency from the registrable body, the Health and Care Professions Council (2022), have recently changed from being vague and taking a noncommittal stance to antiracism to being more direct. Standard 5 states 'recognise the impact of culture, equality and diversity on practice and practise in a non-discriminatory and inclusive manner'; although 'non' should be 'anti', hopefully it's still a work in progress. This emphasis on equality and diversity by the profession has not always worked in favour of the minoritised members because it is not antiracism. The World Federation of Occupational Therapists (WFOT) (2019) appears to promote silence on calling out on issues of injustices, and there appears to be an absence of occupational therapy international dialogue on racism and human rights issues globally. Silence can be construed as acceptance which further perpetuates the maintenance of these social structures of injustice. The Royal College of Occupational Therapists has taken no tangible actions to address this, until recently, due to a campaigning pressure group BAMEOTUK.

AUTHOR'S VOICE: ODETH

I am the only Black occupational therapy member in a team. I remember that no one asked how I was after the murder of George Floyd. Colleagues would be more interested in the rioting and looting stories and 'relished' in pointing out that this was being done by Black people. My white occupational therapy colleagues were not able to identify that their Black colleague was struggling, being re-traumatised with every image and the negative information coming up in the media. My pain was invisible to them and that made me feel a sense of not belonging in the workspace.

Beginning and sustaining antiracism in occupational therapy in the UK

Within occupational therapy in the UK, we have recently started to talk about racism. This is following the death of George Floyd, May

2020, the impact of the pandemic and the pressure from BAMEOTUK Network. The profession refers to being inclusive without acknowledging that people and communities from BAME populations continue to be excluded. Critical race theory advocates that racism is a social construct and racism is an everyday accepted truth (Delgado & Stefancic 2017). There is a requirement to admit that racism leads to occupational injustice which must be called out (Simaan 2020b). As occupational therapists, if we are going to deliver on our professional principles of person-centredness, inclusion and occupational justice, it is necessary that we visibly demonstrate practice and deliver services that are culturally responsive and ethnorelative. In doing so, we disrupt and diminish the influence of white centric hegemonies and structures that continue the status quo of institutional racism in occupational therapy and its hosting organisations.

Racial injustice is often rooted in institutions; hence, we need to ensure that antiracism and equity are embedded in our processes and policies systemically. 'Occupational therapists around the world are obligated to promote occupational rights as the actualization of human rights' (World Federation of Occupational Therapists 2019: 2). According to Grullon *et al.* (2018), occupational injustice occurs when participation in occupation is barred, confined, segregated or restricted; this is the life experiences of majority BAME populations in the UK due to institutional racism. Leaders must show a willingness to listen to the lived experience of their BAME staff/members and service users, and act on what they hear. There must be willingness to examine policies and procedures and balance these alongside the lived experience of their members/employees and service users to bring about meaningful change. 'The cyclical nature between processes [e.g. within occupational therapy process] and outcomes [e.g. racial health disparities in mental health services] of social injustice create a self-perpetuating phenomenon. Like a virus, social injustice infects the host system from individuals to families to institutions' (Jemal 2017: 604). Fundamentally, this change starts with the leaders and board members of the institutions that train, hire and govern occupational therapists. They have an essential role to change the culture that enables institutional racism. Leaders need to act in allyship, collaborating with their BAME service users and occupational therapists to start the antiracist change.

Alongside leaders, individual occupational therapists must hold themselves to account to practise antiracist occupational therapy through, for example, critical reflection, responding to BAME service user feedback, engagement in learning antiracist and equitable ways of working, unlearning white supremacy, disrupting inequitable policies and practices, becoming political, all as evidence of an ongoing active process and commitment to antiracism, equity and justice. The professional community needs to show solidarity with their peers of BME backgrounds and must come together as collective collaboratives to deliver antiracist occupational therapy.

Issues of Brazil

Brazil, whose genesis is based on the slave trade, slavery and the servile regime, developed a process of racism that remains rooted in the daily lives of Black people to this day. Racism is a social phenomenon that structures and permeates social relations, but it presents itself in society in a veiled way, such that in daily life we do not readily identify the racist situations that people suffer.

In Brazil, the idea of racial democracy is still emphasised – the tropical paradise of democratic co-existence of races (Fernandes 1989) – even though it becomes clear that the racial issue marks socio-economic and rights inequality, thus establishing the existence of racism that permeates this social dynamic. It is a 'society that lives with thousands of situations of racism in its daily lives and ignores, minimizes and ends up leaving an ethical gap, with perverse effects for the whole Black population' (Santos 2013: 76). The Black populations live daily with systemic practices of racism in their various occupations, which creates difficulty for Black individuals, and privileges the white people. This is a whole cultural framework based on the racial hierarchy, which legitimises the practice of institutionalised racism. The outcomes from the systemic persistent impact of racism on the existence of these populations, modify their biochemistry (Williams 2016) and life circumstances so that they become ill and add to the statistics on the increasing lower life expectancy of this population (Santos 2013). Thus, we can understand the harms from the impact of racism on the individuals' constitutions as well as their ability to participate in their social occupations. Amorim *et al.* (2020) summarises the impact of racism on Black lives by stating that a racialised society is configured to benefit the white person shaped by racism.

According to Farias *et al.* (2018) and Farias & Lopes (2020), based on the understanding of these problems in Brazil, it is vital to see the occupational therapist functioning as social articulator, placing themselves as an agent who is politically and ethically committed to delivering antiracist practice. Amorim *et al.* (2020) points out that in the practice of occupational therapists in Brazil, the profession deals daily with the Black population, especially because they are in public institutions and services, which serve a greater number of Black people. However, this did not trigger the Brazilian occupational therapists to include this cultural aspect in their research and practices; more likely it is usually an afterthought in the process. More focus is needed in the literature on the historical and current reality of national Blackness, to understand more specifically aspects of African-Brazilian cultural expression and the daily lives of the subjects involved in this dynamic. In this sense, Farias & Lopes (2020) indicate that, in general it is perceived that the debates, research and actions of occupational therapy with the Black population are still in development in Brazil and in the world. However, it is important to recognize and value these collaborations as enablers of some forward movement, even though small and slow, to search for a technical-political antiracist praxis.

Some of the advances in the debate in the Brazilian scene can be read in the Editorial "Social asphyxias" of black population and issues for occupational therapy' (Amorim *et al.* 2020). The authors argue that the debates began to be promoted more latently within the profession from national and international events such as:

- the COVID-19 pandemic, which has exposed social and racial inequality in Brazil and in the world, the BAME populations being more exposed to the disease and with fewer resources for prevention and treatment

- the demonstrations led by the Black Lives Matter movement, following the murder of George Floyd, which began in the United States and expanded to several countries, including Brazil

- the demonstrations and debates in Brazil against the genocide of Black children and young people, which occurred after the atrocity of the death of the boy Miguel, a Black five-year-old son of a maid, who fell from the building of his mother's employers, due to the negligence of the white employer. This incident rekindled the historical problem of the genocide of Black children and young people in Brazil.

Thus, from these tragic events of injustices and inhumanity, the issues of the Black population for Brazilian occupational therapy are gaining more attention, strengthening the position of those who have already been doing work in this area despite them being few and working from the macro-social perspective for the profession to place themselves as agents that are not neutral within a society structured by racism.

Some movements have pushed the antiracist debate, causing controversy and provoking the profession to act. We have seen the construction of an Anti-Racist Manifesto of Brazilian occupational therapy, built by several professional bodies in some parts of the country; the Association of Occupational Therapy of the State of São Paulo also built a manifesto on the theme, launching the campaign #TerapiaOcupacionalAntirracista. The Brazilian Association of Occupational Therapists released a Manifesto Note #VidasNegrasImportam, in defence of the struggle of the Black population from a critical-reflexive and antiracist occupational therapy position (Amorim *et al.* 2020).

In addition, Black occupational therapists have been called to develop spaces for dissemination and training on the theme of ethnic-racial relations and occupational therapy. Ambrosio *et al.* (2020) in their research identified that, in 2020, there were only eight virtual debates on antiracism and the Black population.

Furthermore, in Brazil, some groups are mobilising to get together to do more; for example, the Dona Ivone Lara Group: Studies and Research in Occupational Therapy and Black Population, which consists of young black occupational therapists, and the Group of Studies AFETO (Africanities and Feminisms: Education and Occupational Therapy), in which students and professionals of occupational therapy and education consider studies on antiracist and antipatriarchal practices among other groups (Amorim *et al.* 2020).

Finally, it is worth highlighting once again how the COVID-19 pandemic is affecting the Black population in Brazil, and how this is further showing the status quo based on injustices involving racial, social and health inequalities. Although this occurred worldwide, Farias and Leite Junior (2021) and Santos *et al.* (2020) point out that in

Brazil, the Black population is the most vulnerable in this context, being more exposed to death, due to socio-economic disadvantage. Moreover, this population does not have access to social rights, including health services, or access to education, social protection, adequate housing, basic sanitation services, internet, employment, income and more, which are factors for social determinants of health and wellbeing. The issues are the outcomes of institutional racism which existed before the pandemic. According to Farias and Leite Junior (2021), this scenario triggered by inequality will worsen in the post-pandemic context, and therefore requires occupational therapists to think about an agenda for this new context – one that aims to disrupt racial inequalities. Thus, there is an urgent need to build and strengthen policies that address the specificities of the different social groups in these inequitable situations (Farias & Leite Junior 2021). As Malfitano *et al.* (2020: 403) state, equality:

> ...in the everyday life of all people only happens if we advocate for a possible quality of life for all, considering differences and power, which bring meaning and to life. If we assume the fight to reduce inequalities, it necessarily involves the advocacy for social security and our professional role in this field.

Thoughts on how Brazil and the UK can create an antiracist occupational therapy profession

From the exposed realities, there are some advancements from recognising the consequences of the unequal race relations around the world. Groups of occupational therapists have been calling for re-evaluation of the theoretical and methodological structures of the profession, including the various sub-areas and perspectives. It is understood that these movements take place in some axes under certain topics of debate, including the following:

- Revisiting the historical paths of the profession and overcoming a neutral perspective in the face of racism and social problems, understanding that therapeutic-occupational action is always technical and political (Barros *et al.* 2002; Barros *et al.* 2005; Lopes & Malfitano 2020; Farias & Lopes 2020; Freire 1987, 2013), which has been affirmed by the Brazilian social occupational therapy. This includes admitting the historical neglect of this professional group in relation to racial issues, and from there starting to think about ways to position and operationalize antiracist practices from collective work with peers and representative institutions.

- (Re)formulating and developing theories surrounding occupational therapy know-how at a national and global level, in dialogue with critical race theories, with the aim of building knowledge dialogues to understand these issues in a macro and micro-social way, within a socio-historical and cultural context.

- Involving the initial and continuous training of occupational therapists, which puts these themes in evidence so that they have knowledge and resources to formulate practices that do not reproduce racial inequalities, but affirm the right for Black populations to live and thrive. For example, we need to incorporate history and sociology about racism and institutional racism into the curricula of occupational therapy courses. We need professionals to recognize themselves as agents who must stand up to institutional racism, avoiding the maintenance of racial inequality.

- Formulating strategies, resources and technologies for carrying out work in the various services that involves monitoring and daily intervention, with the technical and political commitment of awareness-raising practices. From the movement of practical and theoretical professional reformulation, we can inform the lens of occupational therapy to promote justice.

- Having committed leaders, professional bodies and council representatives of occupational therapy to carry out this work on antiracism. Permanent agendas are needed that foster strategies and policies to allow the practice of occupational therapy to be antiracist; for example, raising the debate and discussions on the topic, seeking training in antiracism as therapists, services or organisations, identifying or creating funding for research on antiracism and occupational therapy.

It is vital to understand that an occupational therapist should be a social advocate for antiracism (Barros *et al.* 2005; Barros *et al.* 2007), to produce spaces, activities and moments of debate and dialogue in favour of not (re) producing stigmas, discrimination and racism across the practices of occupational therapy in the various services in mental health, physical rehabilitation, the hospital context, the social context and the school context.

The paths to this can be exemplified in a practice carried out by one of the authors of this chapter.

AUTHOR'S VOICE: MAGNO

I was invited with an occupational therapist, together with a professional psychologist, to carry out a group activity at a public Brazilian university. The objective was to discuss institutional racism and ways of coping, with young Black and non-Black individuals from the university.

This activity then demanded from me, as an occupational therapist, the search for references to understand the categories of racism, especially institutional racism, highlighted by a collection of authors who discuss this theme.

Furthermore, the challenge was to think about ways to work with these themes, and a dynamic called the Walk of Privileges was used. The objective was to trigger debates on the themes about the privileges of the white population in society, and especially in the university.

This activity required management to carry out awareness processes, especially for Black youth, and to welcome and empower Black youth.

Thus, this practice was only possible from the assimilation of demand and the search for information, placing occupational therapy as an agent of the debate.

The occupational therapy profession must demonstrate commitment to antiracist practice and engage in antiracist strategising systemically

As Paulo Freire (2013, 1979) reminds us, it is essential to understand the professional commitment, which involves a human being's own commitment, to contribute to processes of humanisation and transformation of oppressive realities (Farias & Lopes 2020). Ahmed-Landeryou *et al.* (2022) suggest developing antiracist occupational therapy from a decolonial approach through deep interrogation of self, profession and practice. Bearing this in mind, for occupational therapists, within their historical commitment to widen the possibilities for those who have barriers in daily living, it is important to understand and position themselves against racial issues. For in denying this, there is a danger of reproducing processes of subordination. Therefore, adhering to key concepts in the profession relating to ethical-political-antiracist commitment is essential.

> In the key to the ethical-political commitment, we assumed to overcome the neutrality bias, understanding that the conditions of power that generate social exclusion are the result of social relationships woven and for structural inequality and political options. (Farias & Lopes 2020: 1350)

The action to take is centred on social justice (Freire 1979; Farias & Lopes 2020), essential for a profession and its activities that take place in the world and seek to contribute to the survival of humanity, based on personal and social emancipation for Black individuals, which will benefit all individuals who do not identify as Black.

The pandemic has taught us that change is inevitable. Change instils hope for a re-imagined better way of being and for society, or change can cause fear, for the path is unknown and so are the consequences and outcomes. Change can be a slow burn or a rapid restructuring. However, in our lives change is a constant feature (Graham 2019), and eventually we all have to engage with it if we are going to make just and equitable progress for communities.

In light of recent events, the time has come for us as a global occupational therapy profession to embrace antiracist change and take action. We must start to dismantle the structures that perpetuate inequity and racism within the profession. This will require revised strategies on all fronts to combat institutional racism:

- Occupational therapy leaders must understand how they can use their privilege to enact antiracist and equity change. They must listen to the voices of the marginalised and minoritised, the very people who are experiencing racism and inequity, and collaborate with them to shape impactful change and be held to account.

- Occupational therapy professional institutions must first

acknowledge their part in enabling the status quo of institutional racism, before they can honestly work in conjunction to address the structural inequities that exist within the profession and wider system.

- Occupational therapy education institutions must decolonise the curriculum, shaping it by centring the voices of Black and global majority student populations, and integrating content about the history of racism, equity, social justice, culture, belonging and power, and their influence on and ability to disrupt race inequalities and health disparities. A whole curriculum approach is needed, with human rights as a core tenet.

- The occupational therapy profession, professional bodies and regulators must collect data to monitor and evaluate the impact of just change. Data must be used to drive improvements and to ensure accountability for antiracist change, and not just as a source for inactively quoting.

- Occupational therapy leaders and boards must 'walk the talk' and model the behaviours for antiracist culture change. They must put money and resources behind the change they expect from others.

- Occupational therapy selection and recruitment processes, for employment or admission to university, must be based on evidenced-informed, fair and transparent principles, and provide regular accumulatively developmental training for staff, regarding antiracism, cultural humility and justice. Paperwork should be reviewed to ensure it is fit for antiracist purposes. Again, data must be collected to monitor and evaluate changes.

- Occupational therapy organisations, service and courses must prioritise psychological safety and cultural responsiveness to support staff to integrate this in work and enable the reporting of racism or complaints/whistleblowing regarding racism as another tool for learning and collecting data for change, rather than fearing it.

- Occupational therapy should celebrate the diversity of thoughts and opinions that come with a diverse workforce. A diverse team has the benefit of performing better and being effectively responsive by being creative and innovative away from the traditional solutions.

- Occupational therapy must nurture a culture of responsibility and develop systems of measures in situ to hold the organisation accountable for antiracism, anti-discrimination, equity and diversity changes and performance activities.

Ending thoughts

In this chapter, we exposed two realities with different specificities, which may have made some dialogues difficult. However, our objectives here were not to provide fixed answers on the subject, but to share reflections to enable you to think of context-specific possibilities for you to practise anti-oppressive, anti-discriminatory and antiracist occupational therapy.

The task is ample and complex, but we believe that we already have the principles and knowledge to start the work; we just have to care a damn to start.

Examples of next steps you could take to develop the profession and your antiracist occupational therapy practice (add to the list as you develop yourself further)

We want to end the chapter with ideas for next steps, to highlight that antiracism work is not an endpoint but a continuous process. We hope that this book will be the springboard to help you to be actively and continuously antiracist in occupational therapy and beyond. Perera and Douglas (2020) advise that occupational therapists must be accountable for their individual learning (and unlearning) and look for ways of changing themselves and practising as a collective professional group.

Otto Scharmer's (2015) four levels of better listening – learn to apply the fourth level. Have you any other frameworks that could help you develop your antiracism action?

Table 9.1: Otto Scharmer's four levels of listening for leaders and therapists

Level 1: Downloading	Using old habits and patterns of listening	Listening to reconfirm what you believe you know already: 'I know that already'
Level 2: Factual listening	Open mind – listening from outside	Noticing that there is new or different information/data that can be added to what you know already: 'That's new to me'
Level 3: Empathetic listening	Open heart – listening from within	Starting to see and respect the other person's perspective and connecting relationally with that person: 'I can see and understand where you're coming from'
Level 4: Generative listening	Open will – listening from the source	Envisioning a different better/ best future and investing in making it emerge, without one's ego and prejudices/biases getting in the way. Letting go and sharing your power and privilege: 'This is about something bigger than me that I feel connected to'

Safe, active national and international spaces – why do we need these spaces for BIPOC/BAME populations and what are we going to do to support these spaces? This is a call to action for a global resource to be purposefully put aside for regular gatherings of those most affected by racism – paid for by those who benefit from racism. BAME/BIPOC occupational therapy student and staff populations need to get together – we need to meet, talk, share, listen, strategise and plan. There must be no more just talking about the racial wounds and asking white people to reflect. Our next steps must look very different from today. BAME/BIPOC occupational therapy staff and students will not engage in discussions of anti-oppression, equity or antiracism if the space is not open, welcoming and secure. If, as occupational therapists we don't hear from the person, or as Scharmer states, hear the source, how can we start to disrupt the injustices experienced by service users or peers? Terms such as psychological safety (Delizonna 2017) and cultural safety (Lock *et al.* 2021) are mentioned more due to health and career inequity, but these are reform concepts for antracism and inequity. Clarke *et al.* (2016) concluded from their research that those safe therapeutic environments instil hope, enable belonging and are built on mutual trust, relational connection and sharing of power. Perera and Douglas's (2020) blog states that this can be done by 'leaving our assumptions at the door, being present, listening, asking questions and understanding that people experience reality differently from ourselves'.

Education – what are you going to do to enable occupational therapy education to create belonging and to decentre whiteness? Education is key to ensure we sustain antiracist practice within the occupational therapy profession. Our training curricula require an overview at every level to ensure that antiracist teachings are included. There are many authors of antiracist education, such as George J. Sefa Dei, Gus John, Heidi Mirza or Kalwant Bhopal, to name a few, but none are from the occupational therapy profession. We have only a few papers on occupational therapy education, for example Grenier (2020) and Simaan (2020a, 2020b). There appears to be a lack of strategic drive from occupational therapy bodies such as the WFOT or from professional bodies; the leadership, vision and investment is lacking for antiracism to be integrated into the curriculum and shape the delivery of curricula and accountability. There is an urgent need to examine the racial heat map of occupational therapy lecturers and authors of the core literature lists (how many are from BAME/indigenous/minoritised populations, who is delivering what and why?). We need a review and reframing of our models so that they are culturally responsive to not maintaining the status quo of white supremacy, and more. By doing this, we place a critical lens on curricula from equity and justice perspectives, collaboratively with students and lecturers from BAME and indigenous populations. Our training institutions must utilise co-production at each stage when developing and delivering the training programme. These antiracism changes must be monitored and reviewed and must be measurable, and they should include agreed mandatory requirements which are consistent across institutions.

Career development and progression – what are you going to do to enable equitable access to career development, opportunities and progression for occupational therapy staff from BAME/BIPOC heritage backgrounds? The UK Workforce Race Equality Standards report (NHS England 2021) provided data that shows little has changed for BAME staff in the health and social care. Yes, more are passing interviews, but then get stuck in the lower paid jobs. The pandemic also showed that BAME/BIPOC staff in health and social care were the majority who died due to many reasons, for example less likely to speak up about not receiving personal protective equipment or working in unsafe situations in comparison to their white peers (Public Health England 2020a). As occupational therapists, we purport to work under the social justice framework, but this is contradicted if those from BAME/BIPOC populations do not feel that they can be themselves or feel a sense of belonging at work (McGregor-Smith 2017). For example, as a starting point, the Royal College of Occupational Therapists already has a career development framework, and this could be reviewed to ensure that antiracist practice is demonstrated and measured, and that equity and justice are embedded within it.

Leadership – what are you going to do to enable greater representation of leaders from BAME heritage backgrounds? Beagan *et al.* (2022: 59–60) identify as one of their study's key messages: 'Racism is normalized in the profession; racialized occupational therapists experience it at interpersonal, institutional, and structural levels, causing extensive psycho-emotional harm.' Work is needed to ensure the removal of the 'glass ceiling' that exists for BAME staff populations, and which is particularly evident in the NHS (NHS England 2021). Roger Kline (2020), in his *British Medical Journal* leader blog, wrote:

> We know 'stretch opportunities' (acting up, secondments, involvement in projects teams) are the most important contribution to career progression but these are mainly accessed by a 'tap on the shoulder'. Instead insist every 'stretch opportunity' should be filled in a transparent manner utilising a positive action approach.

He directs that these opportunities should not fall on individual BAME staff populations to seek out, but must be readily advertised, promoted and accessible. These opportunities could be offered by the Royal College of Occupational Therapists to support and develop occupational therapists from BAME heritage as secondments for qualified practitioners to attain experience of senior and leadership positions, alongside student placements with the RCOT.

Occupational therapy governing bodies and regulators – how will you collaborate with Black, indigenous and global majority populations to make sure that the agendaos and standards of practice clearly hold accountable your-selves and occupational therapists to demonstrate antiracism, equity and justice? The Health and Care Professions Council (HCPC) has already started action for change in forming an EDI (Equity Diversity Inclusion) forum that meets regularly with a wide stakeholder base, and their first action was to review the language for the standards of proficiency (SoPs) for registrable practice. In autumn 2022, they published the new version of the SoPs that has some focus on the registrant demonstrating anti-discriminatory and culturally aware practice. The language still needs work, but they have actively started changing (Health and Care Professions Council 2022).

The Royal College of Occupational Therapists (RCOT) has taken some tentative steps to explore what they should be doing regarding EDI actions but has not quite fully formed what this would look like. They have a steering group, made of minoritized and marginalized groups, to start to give a steer on where the RCOT should be developing projects and actions.

Both organisations still have lots of work to do in diversifying their own staff populations, which remain currently predominantly white as you go up the ladder. But to start right they need to collaborate with the very populations experiencing minoritisation, marginalisation and othering under occupational therapy.

Resources – what do you know of that are promoting antiracism in occu-pational therapy? Here are a few to get you started:

- BAMEOTUK YouTube channel: www.youtube.com/channel/ UCKobQkHUlolCiXgrvn7lg_A/videos

- DisruptOT: www.disruptot.org

- Article: Cadernos Brasileiros de Terapia Ocupacional. *Brazilian Journal of Occupational Therapy*: www.scielo.br/j/cadbto

- Book: *Social Occupational Therapy* by R. Lopes & A.P.S. Malfi-tano. www.elsevier.com/books/social-occupational-therapy/lopes/978-0-323-69549-7

- Book: *Political Practice in Occupational Therapy* edited by N. Pollard, D. Sakellariou & F. Kronenberg

- Book series: *Occupational Therapy Without Borders*

  - *Learning from the Spirit of Survivors* (first edition) by F. Kronenberg, S.S. Algado & N. Pollard

  - *Towards an Ecology of Occupation-Based Practices* (Vol 2, first edition) by F. Kronenberg, N. Pollard & D. Sakellariou

  - *Integrating Justice With Practice* (second edition) by N. Pollard & D. Sakellariou

- Book: Concepts in Occupational Therapy: Understanding Southern Perspectives by S.A. Dsouza, R. Galvaan & E. Ramugondo. www.exoticindiaart.com/book/details/concepts-in-occupational-therapy-understanding-southern-perspectives-naz744/?sitecurrency=GBP&gclid =EAIaIQobChMIj-6WtZKN_QIVwe7tChoAewv6EAQYASABEgJIKPD_BwE

- Article: Occupational consciousness by E.L. Ramugondo. Journal of Occupational Science. https://doi.org/10.1080/14427591.2015.1042516

- Journal: Occupational Therapy Now, March 2022, special edition: Social Accountability. www.caot.ca/document/7758/OT%20Now_Mar_22.pdf

What else could you add?

Web-based resources

www.kingsfund.org.uk/blog/2019/11/lived-experiences-ethnic-minority-staff-nhs

https://otsforaction.org/otsforactionewsletter/2020/3/28/racism-in-occupational-therapy-why-anti-racist-occupational-therapy-is-the-current-and-forever-work-of-ots

https://rehab.queensu.ca/blog/here-and-now-challenge-occupational-therapists

https://otpotential.com/blog/occupational-therapy-and-racial-injustice

https://pearnkandola.com/diversity-and-inclusion-hub/bias/imposter-syndrome

https://blog.usejournal.com/dear-allies-you-will-be-tired-but-you-must-persist-250fd40ce0e6

https://gottabeot.wordpress.com/2020/05/31/black-ots-matter-changing-your-ot-practice-to-combat-racism-address-racial-trauma-and-promote-healing

www.theguardian.com/commentisfree/2020/jul/26/racism-making-us-ill-prejudice

www.theguardian.com/uk-news/2020/jun/10/be-the-change-20-positive-ways-to-fight-for-a-fairer-world

https://ot-magazine.co.uk/changing-the-face-of-ot

https://blogs.bmj.com/bmjleader/2020/06/13/after-the-speeches-what-now-for-nhs-staff-race-discrimination-by-roger-kline

https://make-it-plain.org/2021/02/12/social-work-is-institutionally-racist-heres-how-we-fix-it

www.hsj.co.uk/leadership/leaders-who-perform-on-racial-inclusion-dont-fool-bame-staff/7023540.article www.linkedin.com/pulse/oops-goes-corporate-knee-jennifer-amen-izekor

Reflective quadrant: Identifying, recording and understanding learning from the chapter

What? (Describe what have I learnt)	**Relevance?** (Why is this topic relevant to me/to my practice? Relate/align to/with, e.g., research literature, professional bodies' proficiencies/competencies, service delivery/service user benefit, legislation – briefly and critically discuss)
How will this learning change me/my practice?	**What actions do I have to follow up on to develop my learning in this area or apply to my practice?** (SMART goal format or similar)

Glossary

BAME: Acronym for Black Asian and Minoritised Ethnicities populations/groups. Some people use it as a noun, such as BAME people, but there is no population that is BAME and it should not be used as such.

BIPOC: Acronym for Black, Indigenous, People of Color populations/groups. A term popular in the USA and Canada.

BME: Acronym for Black Minoritised Ethnicities populations/groups. A term used in the UK.

Colonialism: Occupation of indigenous/native peoples and lands by another country, for economic exploitation and political control. The other country takes over and rules (Ndlovu-Gatsheni 2020).

Coloniality: How colonialism is still currently in play in organisations, policies, laws, knowledge and more.

Cultural safety: Striving to redress the power imbalance from institutional racism and discrimination, in systems and processes, for equality of outcomes for the public, integrating, for example, valuing differences and lived experiences, centring the minoritised and marginalised voices and continuously co-developing actions, building in trust, respect and reciprocity, all this and more, as usual practice.

Decoloniality: Exposing coloniality in structures and organisations through critical evaluations, and developing actions to disrupt and resist it.

Decolonising: Carrying out actions to undo the harms of colonialism. It is political, it is for equity and justice and it involves reparations. For example, instead of land acknowledgements, why not give the land back? It is about economic and climate redress and much more.

Diversity: A range of actors that make up the differences between individuals, communities and societies and account for human behaviour. There are so many that what is listed does not fully cover it: gender, age, heritage, nationality, language, culture, religion, gender, socio-economic class, mental, physical abilities and more (Diller 2015).

Equality of outcomes: The general conditions needed to thrive in society, structurally resourced by government, society in collaboration with communities, whether that be in school, for wages, employment opportunities, healthcare, and so on.

Ethnicity: Originating from the Greek *ethnos* meaning people or nation (Hamer *et al.* 2020), the term is used to assign peoples to a group because of culture (includes e.g. diet, religion) or language or common descent/ancestry (Hamer *et al.* 2020). However, at some unspecified time later it became associated with pagans, othering and minoritising groups (Schaefer 2008; Sekulić 2008). Ethnicity plays a major role in the understanding of health inequalities, racism and social determinants as their interactions result in negative outcomes for the identified populations (Marmot *et al.* 2020a).

Ethnocentric service: A service that is structurally designed to predominantly benefit one group.

Ethnorelative service: A service structurally designed on the principles of equity, justice and cultural safety, to strive towards delivering equality of outcomes for all who use the service.

Gaslighting: Emotional abuse, where the person on the receipt of this starts to question their experienced reality because the person delivering this sets up a false explanation of reality as true.

Health inequalities: 'Health inequalities are avoidable, unfair and systemic differences in health between different groups of people' (Williams *et al.* 2020), resulting, for example in England, in a 19-year difference in the number of years in living healthily between the poorest and wealthiest regions (The Health Foundation 2021). Health inequalities are linked to inequalities in maternal health, early years education, access to food, living wage, access to housing and access to health and social care, caused by systemic racism, discrimination and poverty (Marmot *et al.* 2020a). These are usually influenced by social determinants which consider where people are born and live, their education level, work opportunities and age. Marmot *et al.*'s (2020a) epidemiological report shows that social determinants play a role in influencing our health and wellbeing, but squarely puts the overall cause on systemic racism as most of those who are impacted are from Black, minoritised and marginalised groups.

Health inequities: Health equity is enabling individuals to receive personalised care that will meet their health needs and enable them to thrive. Health inequities are systemic political and economic conditions which disadvantage the marginalized and poor of society. 'Health inequities are differences in health status [relative wellness or illness] or in the distribution of health resources between different population groups, arising from the social conditions in which people are born, grow, live, work and age. Health inequities are unfair and could be reduced by the right mix of government policies' (World Health Organisation 2018).

Imperialism: Where policy/ies of economics and political ideas drive the practice of colonialism.

Inclusion: 'The practice or policy of providing equal access to opportunities and resources for people who might otherwise be excluded or marginalized, such as those who have physical or mental disabilities and members of [minoritised] groups.' (Oxford Dictionary online)

Institutional racism: 'The unfair policies and discriminatory practices of particular institutions (schools, workplaces, etc.) that routinely produce racially inequitable outcomes for people from BME heritages and advantages white people. Individuals within institutions take on the power imbalance of the institution when they reinforce racial inequities.' (CUYAHOGA Arts & Culture n.d.)

Microaggression: Interpersonal racism, from one person towards another, which can occur on a daily basis.

Occupation: Activities of daily living that you need to do to survive or exist in the everyday, and/or want to do to thrive and not just exist.

Occupational therapy: An evidence-based therapy that employs the collaborative use of everyday activities/chores/hobbies as a treatment modality for recovery and wellbeing.

Pedagogy: The theory and method of teaching and learning.

Racism: The 'belief that humans are subdivided into distinct groups that are different in their social behavior and innate capacities and that humans can be ranked as superior or inferior' (Newman 2012: 405). The idea of race as a social construct ultimately loosens it from the biological associations it has held since the 18th century (Guillaumin & O'Callaghan 1980; Saini 2019; Rutherford 2020). Racist ideology and categories are born of the colonialist agenda to legitimise racial capital gains and impose their societal and political proclivities as superior, and the right to validate land domination, the extraction of resources and human rights violations of the indigenous/native peoples (Smedley 1998). Grosfoguel (2016) suggests not using reductionist or compact descriptions of racism as this dilutes the complexity, diversity and intersectional nature of the social construct of racism.

> Racism is a global hierarchy of superiority and inferiority along the line of the human that has been politically, culturally and economically produced and reproduced for centuries by the institutions of the 'capitalist/patriarchal western-centric/Christian-centric modern/colonial world-system' (Grosfoguel 2011 cited in Grosfoguel 2016: 10)

> The people classified above the line of the human are recognized socially in their humanity as human beings and, thus, enjoy access to rights (human rights, civil rights, women rights and/or labor rights), material resources, and social recognition to their subjectivities, identities, epistemologies and spiritualities. The people below the line of the human are considered subhuman or non-human... Racism can be marked by colour, ethnicity, language, culture and/or religion (Grosfoguel 2016: 10).

Kendi (2019) makes it clear that to be racist is to support racism through policy, action or inaction. Hence, it is not enough to be non-racist as this is a passive neutral position and supports continuity of racism; what we need to be as a society is antiracist, taking an active position against racism (Kendi 2019).

Settler colonialism: A structure that perpetuates the elimination of indigenous people and cultures to replace them with a settler society (https://en.wikipedia.org/wiki/Settler_colonialism).

Systemic/Structural racism: The enactment of racism through the laws and regulations of society compounded by many societal factors such as history and ideologies, which then interacts and influences the policies, practices, culture and leadership of organisations.

White supremacy: An ideology that a group, usually racialised as white, believe that they are superior to all other populations, hence should be the dominating group in societies, and racism is a way to preserve the white populations' existence and maintain hierarchy of difference (Kendi 2019). This is said to advantage those racialised as white due to their skin colour, resulting in better healthcare, better access to education and other life opportunities (Razai *et al.* 2021). The ideology is also anti-white when it comes to certain groups, such as the traveller communities (Kendi 2019).

References

Accapadi, M.M. (2007). When white women cry: How white women's tears oppress women of color. *The College Student Affairs Journal*, 26(2): 208–2015. Available at: https://files. eric.ed.gov/fulltext/EJ899418.pdf accessed 28 September 2021

Acosta, K.L. (2020). Racism: A public health crisis. *City & Community*, 19(3): 506–515. doi: https://doi.org/10.1111/cico.12518

Acheson, K. & Schneider-Bean, S. (2019). Representing the Intercultural Development Continuum as a pendulum: Addressing the lived experiences of intercultural competence development and maintenance. *European Journal of Cross-Cultural Competence and Management*, 5(1): 42–61. doi: https://doi.org/10.1504/EJCCM.2019.097826

Adams, F. & Casteleijn, D. (2014). New insights in collective participation: A South African perspective. *South African Journal of Occupational Therapy*, 44(1): 81–87

Adorno, T. (1978). *Minima Moralia: Reflections from Damaged Life*. Frankfurt, Germany: Surkamp Verlag

African American Policy Forum. (2009). *A Primer on Intersectionality*. New York, NY: Columbia Law School

Agho, A.O. & John, E.B. (2017). Occupational therapy and physiotherapy education and workforce in Anglophone sub-Saharan Africa countries. *Human Resources for Health*, 15(1): 1–7. doi: https://doi.org/10.1186/s12960-017-0212-5

Agner, J. (2020). Moving from cultural competence to cultural humility in occupational therapy: A paradigm shift. *American Journal of Occupational Therapy*, 74(4): 7404347010p1–7404347010p7. doi: https://doi.org/10.5014/ajot.2020.038067

Ahmed, A.K. (2020). #RhodesMustFall: How a decolonial student movement in the Global South inspired epistemic disobedience at the University of Oxford. *African Studies Review*, 63(2): 281–303. doi: https://doi.org/10.1017/asr.2019.49

Ahmed-Landeryou, M.J., Emery-Whittington, I., Ivlev, S.R. & Elder, R. (2022). Pause, reflect, reframe: Deep discussion in co-creating a decolonial approach for an antiracist framework in occupational therapy. *Occupational Therapy Now*, March/April, 25(2): 14–16. Available at: https://caot.ca/document/7758/OT%20Now_Mar_22.pdf accessed 10 October 2022

Al Busaidy, N.S.M. & Borthwick, A. (2012). Occupational therapy in Oman: The impact of cultural dissonance. *Occupational Therapy International*, 19(3):154–164. doi: https://doi. org/10.1002/oti.1332

Alcoff, L. (1991). The problem of speaking for others. *Cultural Critique*, 20 (Winter 1991–1992): 5–32. doi: https://doi.org/10.2307/1354221

Aldrich, R.M. & Peters, L. (2019). Using occupational justice as a linchpin of international educational collaborations. *American Journal of Occupational Therapy*, 73(3): 7303205100p1–7303205100p10. doi: https://doi.org/10.5014/ajot.2019.029744

Alexander, M. (2010). *The New Jim Crow: Mass Incarceration in the Age of Colorblindness* (revised edition). New York, NY: New Press

Allen, J. (2010). Improving cross-cultural care and antiracism in nursing education: A literature review. *Nurse Education Today*, 30(4): 314–320. doi: https://doi.org/10.1016/j.nedt.2009.08.007

Allen, T. (2012). *The Invention of the White Race: Racial Oppression and Social Control* (J.B. Perry, ed., Vol. 1). London, New York, NY: Verso

All India Occupational Therapists' Association. (2018). *Occupational Therapy: An Indian Historical Perspective*. Available at: https://aiota.org/otindia accessed 24 May 2021

Almeida, S.L. de (2018). *O que é racismo estrutural?* Belo Horizonte, Brazil: Letramento

Ambrosio, L., Queiroz, A.G., Vital, R.S. & Silva, C. (2020). Terapia Ocupacional e relações étnico-raciais na pandemia: entre apagamentos e visibilidades. In *XVII National Meeting of Professors in Occupational Therapy, Virtual Edition – 2020* (pp.173–175). Brazil. Available at: https://drive.google.com/file/d/1Bp_o1oespyT_8PiOJs6rOenaF4XB6OvK/view accessed 21 December 2021

Amen Izekor, J. (2020). Oops there goes that corporate knee... Available at: www.linkedin.com/pulse/oops-goes-corporate-knee-jennifer-amen-izekor accessed 10 February 2023

American Anthropological Association (AAA). (1998). *Statement on Race*. Available at: www.americananthro.org/ConnectWithAAA/Content.aspx?ItemNumber=2583 accessed 28 September 2021

American Friends Service Committee. (2021). *How to intervene if someone is being harassed*. Available at: www.afsc.org/bystanderintervention accessed 24 June 2022

American Masters. (1989). 'James Baldwin: The Price of the Ticket' documentary. Director, Karen Thorsen

American Occupational Therapy Association. (2014). *FAQs: AOTA Board of Directors' position statement on doctoral-level single point of entry for occupational therapists*. Available at: www.aota.org/AboutAOTA/Get-Involved/BOD/OTD-FAQs.aspx accessed 24 June 2022

American Occupational Therapy Association. (2020). Occupational Therapy Practice Framework: Domain and Process—fourth edition. *American Journal of Occupational Therapy*, 74(2): 7412410010p1–7412410010 p.87. doi: https://doi.org/10.5014/ajot.2020.74S2001

American Occupational Therapy Association. (2021). *History of AOTA accreditation*. Available at: www.aota.org/education-careers/accreditation/overview/history.aspx accessed: 26 June 2017

Amorim, S.G., Martins, S., Leite Junior, J.D. & Farias, M.N. (2020). 'Asfixias sociais' da população negra e questões para a Terapia Ocupacional ['Social asphyxias' of black population and issues for occupational therapy]. *Revista Interinstitucional Brasileira de Terapia Ocupacional – Revisbrato*, 4(5): 719–733. doi: https://doi.org/10.47222/2526-3544.rbto36144

Anderson, L.W. & Krathwohl, D.R. (2001). *A Taxonomy for Learning, Teaching, and Assessing: A Revision of Bloom's Taxonomy of Educational Objectives*. London: Longman

Andersen, L.T. & Reed, K.L. (2017). *The History of Occupational Therapy, The 1st Century*. Thorofare, NJ: Slack Incorporated

Angell, A.M. (2014). Occupation-centered analysis of social difference: Contributions to a socially responsive occupational science. *Journal of Occupational Science*, 21(2): 104–116. doi: https://doi.org/10.1080/14427591.2012.711230

Arday, J. (2015). Creating Space and Providing Opportunities for BAME 40 Academics in Higher Education. In C. Alexander & J. Arday (eds), *Aiming Higher: Race, Inequality and Diversity in the Academy* (pp.4–42). London: Runnymede Trust

Arday, J., Belluigi, D.Z. & Thomas, D. (2020). Attempting to break the chain: Reimaging inclusive pedagogy and decolonizing the curriculum within the academy. *Educational Philosophy and Theory*, 53(3): 298–313. doi: https://doi.org/10.1080/00131857.2020.1773257

Association for Project Management. (2022). *What is governance?* Available at: www.apm.org.uk/resources/what-is-project-management/what-is-governance accessed 22 June 2022

Bambra, C., Riordan, R., Ford, J. & Matthews, F. (2020). The COVID-19 pandemic and health inequalities. *Journal of Epidemiology Community Health*, 74: 964–968. Available at: https://jech.bmj.com/content/74/11/964 accessed 15 October 2021

Bailliard, A. (2016). Justice, difference, and the capability to function. *Journal of Occupational Science*, 23(1): 3–16. doi: https://doi.org/10.1080/14427591.2014.957886

References

BAMEOTUK. (2020). *Open letter from BAMEOTUK to RCOT*. Available at: www.rcot.co.uk/ news/rcot-response-open-letter accessed 12 December 2021

Barros, D.D., Ghirardi, M.I.G. & Lopes, R.E. (2002). Terapia ocupacional social. *Revista De Terapia Ocupacional Da Universidade De São Paulo*, 13(3): 95-103. doi: https://doi. org/10.11606/issn.2238-6149.v13i3p95-103

Barros, D.D., Ghirardi, M.I.G. & Lopes, R.E. (2005). Social Occupational Therapy: A Socio-Historical Perspective. In F. Kronenberg, S.S. Algado & N. Pollard (eds), *Occupational Therapy Without Borders: Learning from the Spirit of Survivors* (pp.140-151). Edinburgh: Elsevier Churchill Livingstone

Barros, D.D., Lopes, R.E. & Galheigo, S.M. (2007). Terapia ocupacional social: concepções e perspectivas. In A. Cavalcanti, & C. Galvão (eds), *Terapia Ocupacional - Fundamentação e Prática* (pp.347-353). Rio de Janeiro, Brazil: Guanabara Koogan

Bass-Haugen, J.D. (2009). Health disparities: Examination of evidence relevant for occupational therapy. *American Journal of Occupational Therapy*, 63(1): 24-34. doi: https://doi. org/10.5014/ajot.63.1.24

Batty, D. (2019). Universities failing to address thousands of racist incidents. *The Guardian*. Available at: www.theguardian.com/world/2019/oct/23/universities-failing-to-address-thousands-of-racist-incidents accessed 1 June 2021

Beagan, B.L. (2018). A Critique of Cultural Competence: Assumptions, Limitations, and Alternatives. In C. Frisby & W. O'Donohue (eds), *Cultural Competence in Applied Psychology* (pp.123-138). Cham, Switzerland: Springer

Beagan, B.L. (2020). Commentary on racism in occupational science. *Journal of Occupational Science*, 28(3): 410-413. doi: https://doi.org/10.1080/14427591.2020.1833682

Beagan, B.L. & Chacala, A. (2012). Culture and diversity among occupational therapists in Ireland: When the therapist is the 'diverse' one. *British Journal of Occupational Therapy*, 75(3): 144-151. doi: https://doi.org/10.4276/030802212X13311219571828

Beagan, B.L., Chapman, G.E. & Power, E. (2018). The visible and invisible occupations of food provisioning in low income families. *Journal of Occupational Science*, 25(1): 100-111. doi: https://doi.org/10.1080/14427591.2017.1338192

Beagan, B.L. & Etowa, J. (2009). The impact of everyday racism on the occupations of African Canadian women. *Canadian Journal of Occupational Therapy*, 76(4): 285-293. doi: https:// doi.org/10.1177/000841740907600407

Beagan, B.L., Sibbald, K.R., Bizzeth, S.R. & Pride, T.M. (2022). Systemic racism in Canadian occupational therapy: A qualitative study with therapists. *Canadian Journal of Occupational Therapy*, 89(1): 51-61. doi: 10.1177/00084174211066676

Bell, D. (1973). *Race, Racism and American Law*. Boston, MA: Little and Brown

Bell, D. (1980). Brown v. Board of Education and the interest-convergence dilemma. *Harvard Law Review*, 93(3): 518-533. doi: https://doi.org/10.2307/1340546

Bell, D. (1987). *And We Are Not Saved: The Elusive Quest for Racial Justice*. New York, NY: Basic Books

Bell, D. (1993). *Faces at the Bottom of the Well: The Permanence of Racism*. New York, NY: Basic Books

Bell, D. (2009). Who's Afraid of Critical Race Theory? In E. Taylor, D. Gillborn & G. Ladson-Billings (eds), *Foundations of Critical Race Theory in Education* (pp.37-50). New York, NY: Routledge

Bell, D. (2018). A pedagogical response to decoloniality: Decolonial atmospheres and rising subjectivity. *American Journal of Community Psychology*, 62(3-4): 250-260. doi: https:// doi.org/10.1002/ajcp.12292

Bellis, M.A., Hughes, K., Hardcastle, K., Ashton, K. *et al.* (2013). The impact of adverse childhood experiences on health service use across the life course using a retrospective cohort study. *Journal of Public Health*, 36 (1): 81-91. doi: https://doi.org/10.1177/1355819617706720

Ben, J., Kelly, D. & Paradies, Y. (2020). Contemporary Anti-Racism: A Review of Effective Practice. In J. Solomos (ed.), *Routledge International Handbook of Contemporary Racisms: Contemporary Anti-Racism: A Review of Effective Practice* (pp.205-215). New York, NY: Routledge

Bertrand, M. & Mullainathan, S. (2004). Are Emily and Greg more employable than Lakisha and Jamal? A field experiment on labor market discrimination. *The American Economic Review*, 94(4): 991–1013. doi: https://doi.org/10.1257/0002828042002561

Bhambra, G.K., Gebrial, D. & Nişancıoğlu, K. (2018). *Decolonising the University*. London: Pluto Press

Biko, S. (1978). *I Write What I Like*. London: The Bowerdean Press

Black, R.M. & Wells, S.A. (2007). *Culture Occupation: A Model of Empowerment in Occupational Therapy*. Bethesda, MD: AOTA Press

Blacklivesmatter.com (2020). *Black Lives Matter*. Available at: https://blacklivesmatter.com/about accessed 13 April 2021

Blessett, B. & Littleton, V. (2017). Examining the impact of institutional racism in black residentially segregated communities. *Ralph Bunche Journal of Public Affairs*, 6(1), Article 3. Available at: https://digitalscholarship.tsu.edu/cgi/viewcontent.cgi?article=1032&context=rbjpa accessed 28 September 2021

Bojadžijev, M. (2020). Anti-Racism as Method. In J. Solomos (ed.), *Routledge International Handbook of Contemporary Racisms: Anti-Racism as Method* (pp.193–204). New York, NY: Routledge

Bonilla-Silva, E. (2014). *Racism Without Racists: Color-Blind Racism and the Persistence of Racial Inequality in America* (fourth edition). Lanham, MD: Rowman and Littlefield Publishers

Borrell, C., Espelt, A., Rodríguez-Sanz, M. & Navarro, V. (2007). Politics and health. *Journal of Epidemiology and Community Health*, 61(8): 658–659. doi: https://doi.org/10.1136/jech.2006.059063

Boyt Schell, B.A. & Schell, J.W. (2017). *Clinical and Professional Reasoning in Occupational Therapy*. Philadelphia, PA: Wolters Kluwer

Braveman, B. & Bass-Haugen, J.D. (2009). Social justice and health disparities: An evolving discourse in occupational therapy research and intervention. *American Journal of Occupational Therapy*, 63(1): 7–12. doi: https://doi.org/10.5014/ajot.63.1.7

Braveman, B. & Suarez-Balcazar, Y. (2009). Social justice and resource utilization in a community-based organization: A case illustration of the role of the occupational therapist. *American Journal of Occupational Therapy*, 63(1): 13–23. doi: https://doi.org/10.5014/ajot.63.1.13

Bregman, P. (2012). Diversity training doesn't work. *Harvard Business Review*. Available at: https://hbr.org/2012/03/diversity-training-doesnt-work accessed 8 January 2022

Burke, P.J., Bennett, A., Burgess, C., Gray, K. & Southgate, E. (2016). *Capability, Belonging and Equity in Higher Education: Developing Inclusive Approaches*. Australia: The University of Newcastle Australia

Burgess, Y. (1996). *The Myth of Progress*. Glasgow: Wild Goose Publications

Burkett, K., Morris, E., Manning-Courtney, P., Anthony, J. & Shambley-Ebron, D. (2015). African American families on autism diagnosis and treatment: The influence of culture. *Journal of Autism and Developmental Disorders*, 45(10): 3244–3254. doi: https://doi.org/10.1007/s10803-015-2482-x

Burr, J. (2010). *The Altruistic Self and the Desire of Developing Others: Towards a Post-Development Ethos of Action* [MA thesis]. Nova Scotia, Canada: Dalhousie University

Came, H. (2014). Sites of institutional racism in public health policy making in New Zealand. *Social Science & Medicine*, 106: 214–220. doi: https://doi.org/10.1016/j.socscimed.2014.01.055

Came, H., McCreanor, T., Haenga-Collins, M. & Cornes, R. (2019). Māori and Pasifika leaders' experiences of government health advisory groups in New Zealand. *Kōtuitui: New Zealand Journal of Social Sciences*, 14(1): 126–135. doi: https://doi.org/10.1080/1177083X.2018.1561477

Campbell, C.A. (2019). *From the Slave Ship to Modern Day Lynching in the Streets of America* [MA thesis]. Southern Illinois, USA: University of Edwardsville. Available at: https://media.proquest.com/media/hms/PFT/2/VTsnC?_s=Om7pmSytwMN7JBbno6ulodZgbIM%3D, accessed 16 June 2022

Canadian Association of Occupational Therapists (CAOT). (2011). *CAOT Position Statement: Occupational therapy and cultural safety*. Available at: https://caot.in1touch.org/

References

document/3702/O%20-%20OT%20and%20Cultural%20Safety.pdf accessed 16 October 2022

Cannon, K.G. (2008). Christian imperialism and the transatlantic slave trade. *Journal of Feminist Studies in Religion*, 24(1): 127–134. doi: https://doi.org/10.2979/FSR.2008.24.1.127

Cassidy, J. (1988). Access to health care: A clinician's opinion about ethical issues. *American Journal of Occupational Therapy*, 42: 295–299

Catlin, K. (2021). *Better Allies: Everyday Actions to Create Inclusive, Engaging Workplaces* (S. McGraw, ed.; second edition). USA: Better Allies Press

Center on the Developing Child. (2021). *What are ACEs and how do they relate to toxic stress?* Available at: https://46y5eh11fhgw3ve3ytpwxt9r-wpengine.netdna-ssl.com/wp-content/uploads/2018/08/ACEsInfographic_080218.pdf accessed 24 June 2022

Chan, K., Parikh, M., Thorpe, Jr, R. & Gaskin, D. (2020). Health care disparities in race-ethnic minority communities and populations: Does the availability of health care providers play a role? *Journal of Racial and Ethnic Health Disparities*, 7(3): 539–549. doi: https://doi.org/10.1007/s40615-019-00682-w

Chang, X., Jiang, X., Mkandarwire, T. & Shen, M. (2019). Associations between adverse childhood experiences and health outcomes in adults aged 18–59 years. *PloS One*, 14(2): e0211850. doi: https://doi.org/10.1371/journal.pone.0211850

Charasse-Pouélé, C. & Fournier, M. (2006). Health disparities between racial groups in South Africa: A decomposition analysis. *Social Science & Medicine*, 62(11): 2897–2914. doi: https://doi.org/10.1016/j.socscimed.2005.11.020

Chartered Institute of Personnel and Development (CIPD). (2020). *Diversity and Inclusion in the Workplace*. London: CIPD. Available at: www.cipd.co.uk/knowledge/fundamentals/relations/diversity/factsheet#gref accessed 15 March 2021

Clarke, S., Clarke, J., Brown, R. & Middleton, H. (2016). Hurting and healing in therapeutic environments: How can we understand the role of the relational context? *European Journal of Psychotherapy & Counselling*, 18(4): 1–17. doi: https://doi.org/10.1080/13642537.2016.1260620

Coalition for Racial Equality and Rights (2021). *Introduction to Antiracist Curriculum Development*. Available at: www.crer.scot accessed 15 March 2021

Coghill, Y. (2021). *7 As of Authentic Allyship*. Royal College of Occupational Therapists Conference, Virtual, 30 June

Cole, M. (2021). Understanding Critical Whiteness Studies: Harmful or Helpful in the Struggle for Racial Equity in the Academy? In D.S.P. Thomas & J. Arday (eds), *Doing Equity and Diversity for Success in Higher Education. Palgrave Studies in Race, Inequality and Social Justice in Education* (pp.277–298). Cham, Switzerland: Palgrave Macmillan

Cole, M.B. & Tufano, R. (2020). *Applied Theories in Occupational Therapy: A Practical Approach* (second edition). Thorofare, NJ: Slack Incorporated

Coles, R.L. & Green, C. (eds). (2010). *The Myth of the Missing Black Father*. New York, NY: Columbia University Press

Cook, T., Kursumovic, E. & Lennane, S. (2020). *Exclusive: deaths of NHS staff from COVID-19 analysed*. Available at: www.hsj.co.uk/exclusive-deaths-of-nhs-staff-from-COVID-19-analysed/7027471.article accessed 9 June 2021

Córdoba, G.A. (2020). About new forms of colonization in occupational therapy: Reflections on the idea of occupational justice from a critical-political philosophy perspective. *Cadernos Brasileiros de Terapia Ocupacional*, 28(4): 1365–1381. doi: https://doi.org/10.4322/2526-8910.ctoARF2175

Cornell, D. & Van Marle, K. (2005). Exploring ubuntu: Tentative reflections. *African Human Rights Journal*, 5(2): 195–220. Available at: www.ahrlj.up.ac.za/cornell-d-van-marle-k accessed 24 May 2021

Costa, I.R.B.B. (2021). *A potência dos encontros: contribuições de Yvonne Lara e Elelwani Ramugondo para o campo da terapia ocupacional* [MA thesis]. Brazil: Federal University Fluminense

Costa, M.C., Santos, A.C., Souza, J.V., Costa, J.C., Porto, R.M. & Freire, S.R. (2020). Laboratório ISÉ: construções de estratégias para restituição histórica e existencial de pessoas negras. *Rev. Interinst. Bras. Ter. Ocup. Rio de Janeiro*, 4(5): 734–741. doi: https://doi.org/10.47222/2526-3544.rbto36913

Cousins, S. (2019). *Overcoming Everyday Racism*. London: Jessica Kingsley Publishers

Creek, J. (2010). *The Core Concepts of Occupational Therapy: A Dynamic Framework for Practice*. London: Jessica Kingsley Publishers

Crenshaw, K. (1988). Race, reform, and retrenchment: Transformation and legitimation in antidiscrimination law. *Harvard Law Review*, May 101(7): 1331–1387. doi: https://doi.org/10.2307/1341398

Crenshaw, K. (1989). Demarginalizing the intersection of race and sex: A Black feminist critique of antidiscrimination doctrine, feminist theory and anti-racist politics. *University of Chicago Legal Forum*, 8(1): 139–167. Available at: https://chicagounbound.uchicago.edu/uclf/vol1989/iss1/8 accessed 24 June 2022

Crenshaw, K. (1997). Race, Reform, and Retrenchment: Transformation and Legitimation in Antidiscrimination Law. In N. Gates (ed.), *Critical Race Theory: Essays on the Social Construction of 'Race'* (pp.85–141). New York, NY: Garland Publishing

Crenshaw, K. (2016). *The urgency of intersectionality*. Available at: www.youtube.com/watch?v=akOe5-UsQ2o accessed 5 January 2022

Crenshaw, K. (2017). *On Intersectionality: Essential Writings*. New York, NY: New Press

Crenshaw, K.N., Gotanda, G., Peller, G. & Thomas, K. (eds) (1995). *Critical Race Theory: The Key Writings that Formed the Movement*. New York, NY: The New Press

Crowe, J. (2018). Black Lives Matter to contribute to Chicago Police-Reform Plan. *National Review*. Available at: www.nationalreview.com/2018/03/black-lives-matter-to-contribute-to-chicago-police-reforms accessed 9 June 2021

CUYAHOGA Arts & Culture. (n.d.). *Four levels of racism – Race Forward Model*. Available at: www.cacgrants.org/assets/ce/Documents/2019/FourLevelsOfRacism.pdf accessed 10 February 2023

Dabbah, M. (2014). *What is cultural sensitivity?* Available at: www.redshoemovement.com/what-is-cultural-sensitivity accessed 15 March 2021

Dabiri, E. (2021). *What White People Can Do Next: From Allyship to Coalition*. New York, NY: Harper Perennial

DaCunha, J. (2016). *Disrupting Eurocentric Education through a Social Justice Curriculum*. [MA thesis]. Available at: https://commons.clarku.edu/cgi/viewcontent.cgi?article=1087&context=idce_masters_papers accessed 21 December 2021

Davies, M. (2022). *Chart of the week: The over-representation of Black people as restricted patients in secure hospitals*. London: Nuffield Trust. Available at: www.nuffieldtrust.org.uk/resource/chart-of-the-week-the-over-representation-of-black-people-as-restricted-patients-in-secure-hospitals accessed 18 June 2022

Davis, R. (2016). *Responsibility and Public Services*. Axminster: Triarchy Press

Decolonising SOAS Working Group. (2018). *Decolonising SOAS Learning and Teaching Toolkit for Programme and Module Convenors*. London: SOAS, University of London

Dei, G.J.S. (1996). *Anti-racism Education, Theory and Practice*. Halifax, Nova Scotia: Fernwood Publishing

Delgado, R. (1995). *Critical Race Theory: The Cutting Edge*. Philadelphia, PA: Templeton University Press

Delgado, R. & Stefancic, J. (2017). *Critical Race Theory: An Introduction*. New York, NY: New York University Press

Delizonna, L. (2017). High-performing teams need psychological safety. Here's how to create it. *Harvard Business Review*, 24 August. Available at: https://hbr.org/2017/08/high-performing-teams-need-psychological-safety-heres-how-to-create-it accessed 10 January 2022

Devakumar, D., Selvarajah, S., Shannon, G., Muraya, K. *et al.* (2020). Racism, the public health crisis we can no longer ignore. *The Lancet*, 395(10242): e112–e113. doi: https://doi.org/10.1016/S0140-6736(20)31371-4

Dhanda, M. (2009). Understanding disparities in student attainment: What do black and minority ethnic students say? Paper presented at the *Annual Meeting of the ISPP 32nd Annual Scientific Meeting*, Trinity College, Dublin, Ireland, 14 July

References

DiAngelo, R. (2018). *White Fragility: Why It's So Hard For White People to Talk About Racism*. New York, NY: Beacon Press

Dickie, V.A. (2004). Culture is tricky: A commentary on culture emergent in occupation. *American Journal of Occupational Therapy*, 58(2): 169–173. doi: https://doi.org/10.5014/ajot.58.2.169

Dike, P. (2013). *The Impact of Workplace Diversity on Organizations* (PhD thesis). Finland: ARCADA University of Applied Sciences. Available at: https://core.ac.uk/download/pdf/38093915.pdf accessed 15 March 2021

Diller, J.V. (2015). *Cultural Diversity: A Primer for the Human Services* (fifth edition). Stamford, CT: Cengage Learning

Dobbin, F. & Kalev, A. (2018). Why doesn't diversity training work? The challenge for industry and academia. *Anthropology Now*, 10(2): 48–55. doi: https://doi.org/10.1080/19428200.2018.1493182

Dobbin, F., Kalev, A. & Kelly, E. (2007). Diversity management in corporate America. *Contexts*, 6(4): 21–27. doi: https://doi.org/10.1525/ctx.2007.6.4.21

Dougall, D. & Buck, D. (2021). *My role in tackling health inequalities: A framework for allied health professionals*. London: The King's Fund. Available at: www.kingsfund.org.uk/publications/tackling-health-inequalities-framework-allied-health-professionals accessed 9 March 2022

Douglas, D., Chrisafis, A. & Modhin, A. (2021). One year on, how George Floyd's murder has changed the world. *The Guardian*, 22 May 2021. Available at: www.theguardian.com/us-news/2021/may/22/george-floyd-murder-change-across-world-blm accessed 9 March 2022

Dowers, E., White, C., Kingsley, J. & Swenson, R. (2019). Transgender experiences of occupation and the environment: A scoping review. *Journal of Occupational Science*, 26(4): 496–510. doi: https://doi.org/10.1080/14427591.2018.1561382

Duncan, E.A.S. (2020). *Foundations for Practice in Occupational Therapy*. Edinburgh: Elsevier

Durocher, E., Gibson, B.E. & Rappolt, S. (2014). Occupational justice: A conceptual review. *Journal of Occupational Science*, 21(4): 418–430. doi: https://dx.doi.org/10.1080/14427591.2013.775692

Eddo-Lodge, R. (2018). *Why I'm No Longer Talking to White People About Race*. London: Bloomsbury Publishing

Edmonson, A.C. & Roloff, K.S. (2008). Overcoming Barriers to Collaboration: Psychological Safety and Learning in Diverse Teams. In E. Salas, G.F. Goodwing, C.S. Burke, *Team Effectiveness in Complex Organizations: Cross Disciplinary Perspectives and Approaches* (pp.217–242). New York, NY: Routledge/Taylor and Francis Group

Edwards, L. (2016). Homogeneity and inequality: School discipline inequality and the role of racial composition. *Social Forces*, 95(1): 55–76. doi: https://doi.org/10.1093/sf/sow038

Elliot, J. (2020). Bryan Knight interview Prof. Jane Elliot 'One Race', 27 June. Available at: www.youtube.com/watch?v=6jM4f9GUFmA accessed 15 March 2021

Emery-Whittington, I. & Te Maro, B. (2018). Decolonising occupation: Causing social change to help our ancestors rest and our descendants thrive. *New Zealand Journal of Occupational Therapy*, 65(1): 12–19

Emery-Whittington, I.G. (2021). Occupational justice – colonial business as usual? Indigenous observations from Aotearoa New Zealand. *Canadian Journal of Occupational Therapy*, 88(2): 153–162. doi: https://doi.org/10.1177/00084174211005891

Fanon, F. (2004). *The Wretched of the Earth*. France: Francois Maspero

Farias, M.N. & Leite Junior, J.D. (2021). Social vulnerability and COVID-19: Considerations based on social occupational therapy. *Cadernos Brasileiros de Terapia Ocupacional*, 29(e2099): 1–13. doi: https://doi.org/10.1590/2526-8910.ctoEN2099

Farias, M.N., Leite Junior, J.D. & Amorim, S.G.S. (2020). Por uma formação e prática antirracista. *Revista Chilena de Terapia Ocupacional*, 20(2): 237–247. doi: https://doi.org/10.5354/0719-5346.2020.54658

Farias, M.N., Leite Junior, J.D. & Costa, I.R.B.B. (2018). Terapia ocupacional e população negra: possibilidades para o enfrentamento do racismo e desigualdade racial (Occupational Therapy and black population: Possibilities for confrontation of racism and racial inequality). *Revista Interinstitutional Brasileira de Terapia Ocupacional*, 2(1): 228–243. doi: https://doi.org/10.47222/2526-3544.rbto1271

Farias, M.N. & Lopes, R.E. (2020). Social occupational therapy: Formulations by Freirean references. *Cadernos Brasileira de Terapia Ocupacional*, 28(4): 1346–1356

Farias, L. & Simaan, J. (2020). Introduction to the Anti-Racism Virtual Issue of the Journal of Occupational Science. *Journal of Occupational Science*, 27(4): 454–459. doi: https://doi.org/10.1080/14427591.2020.1824567

Fernandes, F. (1989). *Significado do Protesto Negro*. São Paulo, Brazil: Cortez Editora

Fernando, S. (2017). *Institutional Racism in Psychiatry and Clinical Psychology: Race Matters in Mental Health*. London: Palgrave Macmillan

Fijal, D. & Beagan, B.L. (2019). Indigenous perspectives on health: Integration with a Canadian model of practice. *Canadian Journal of Occupational Therapy*, 86(3): 220–231. doi: https://doi.org/10.1177/0008417419832284

Finlayson, M.C. (2013). Muriel Driver Memorial Lecture: Embracing our role as change agents. *Canadian Journal of Occupational Therapy*, 80(4): 205–214. doi: https://doi.org/10.1177/0008417413499505

Foucault, M. (1970). *Order of Things: An Archaeology of Human Sciences*. London: Pantheon Books

Frank, G. & Muriithi, B.A.K. (2015). Theorising social transformation in occupational therapy: The American Civil Rights Movement and South African struggle against apartheid as 'occupational reconstructions'. *South African Journal of Occupational Therapy*, 45(1): 11–19

Freeman, T.M., Anderman, L.H. & Jensen, J.M. (2007). Sense of belonging in college freshmen at the classroom and campus levels. *The Journal of Experimental Education*, 75(3): 203–220. doi: https://doi.org/10.3200/JEXE.75.3.203-220

Freire, P. (1972). *Pedagogy of the Oppressed*. New York, NY: Continuum

Freire, P. (1979). *Educação e Mudanç* (12th edition). Rio de Janeiro, Brazil: Paz e Terra

Freire, P. (1987). *Pedagogy of the Oppressed* (17th edition). Rio de Janeiro, Brazil: Paz e Terra

Freire, P. (1993). *Pedagogy of the Oppressed*. London: Penguin Random House Publishing

Freire, P. (2013). *À Sombra Desta Mangueira* (11th edition). Rio de Janeiro, Brazil: Paz e Terra

Friedman, C. & VanPuymbrouck, L. (2021). Ageism and Ableism: Unrecognized Biases in Occupational Therapy Students. *Physical and Occupational Therapy in Geriatrics*, 39(4): 354–369. doi: https://doi.org/10.1080/02703181.2021.1880531

Galvaan, R., Peters, L., Smith, T., Brittain, M. *et al.* (2015). Employers' experiences of having a live-in domestic worker: Insights into the relationship between privilege and occupational justice. *South African Journal of Occupational Therapy*, 45(1): 41–46. doi: http://dx.doi.org/10.17159/2310-3833/2015/v45no1a7

Gandhi-Luthuli Documentation Centre, UKZN. (n.d.). *Apartheid Legislation in South Africa.* Available at: https://scnc.ukzn.ac.za/doc/hist/apartheid%20legislation%20in%20south%20africa.htm accessed 12 April 2021

Gardiner, T., Abraham, S., Clymer, O., Rao, M. & Gnani, S. (2021). Racial and ethnic health disparities in healthcare settings. *British Medical Journal*, 372: n605. doi: https://doi.org/10.1136/bmj.n605

Garza, A. (2014). A herstory of the #BlackLivesMatter movement. *The Feminist Wire*, 7 October . Available at: https://thefeministwire.com/2014/10/blacklivesmatter-2 accessed 15 October 2021

Gee, G.C. & Ford, C.L. (2011). Structural racism and health inequities: Old issues, new directions. *Du Bois Review: Social Science Research on Race*, 8(1): 115–132. doi: https://doi.org/10.1017/S1742058X11000130

George, A. (2018). *The 1968 Kerner Commission Got It Right, But Nobody Listened*. Washington, DC: Smithsonian Magazine. Available at: www.smithsonianmag.com/smithsonian-institution/1968-kerner-commission-got-it-right-nobody-listened-180968318 accessed 18 June 2022

Geronimus, A.T., Hicken, M., Keene, D. & Bound. J. (2006). 'Weathering' and age patterns of allostatic load scores among Blacks and whites in the United States. *American Journal of Public Health*, 96(5): 826–833. doi: https://doi.org/10.2105/ajph.2004.060749

References

Gibson, C. (2020). When the river runs dry: Leadership, decolonization and healing in occupational therapy. *New Zealand Journal of Occupational Therapy*, 67(1): 11–20. Available at: https://go.gale.com/ps/i.do?id=GALE%7CA628283412&sid=google-Scholar&v=2.1&it=r&linkaccess=abs&issn=11710462&p=AONE&sw=w&userGroupName=anon%7Ec467df24 accessed 10 March 2023

Gillborn, D. (1998). Racism, selection, poverty and parents: New Labour, old problems? *Journal of Education Policy*, 13(6): 717–735. doi: https://doi.org/10.1080/0268093980130604

Gillborn, D. (2007). Critical race theory and education: Racism and antiracism in educational theory and praxis. *Discourse: Studies in the Cultural Politics of Education*, 27(1): 11–32. doi: https://doi.org/10.1080/01596300500510229

Gillborn, D. (2011). Once Upon a Time in the UK: Race, Class, Hope and Whiteness in the Academy: Personal Reflections on the Birth of 'BritCrit'. In K. Hylton, A. Pilkington, P. Warmington & S. Housee (eds), *Atlantic Crossings: International Dialogues on Critical Race Theory* (pp.21–38). Birmingham: C-SAP

Gilmore, R.W. (2007). *Golden Gulag: Prisons, Surplus, Crisis, and Opposition in Globalizing California*. Berkeley, CA: University of California Press

Golden, B. (2021). How adverse childhood experiences (ACEs) impact adult anger. *Psychology Today*, 6 June. Available at: www.psychologytoday.com/us/blog/overcoming-destructive-anger/202106/how-adverse-childhood-experiences-aces-impact-adult-anger accessed 14 December 2020

Golos, A. & Tekuzener, E. (2019). Perceptions, expectations and satisfaction levels of occupational therapy students prior to and after practice placement and comparison of practice placement models. *BMC Medical Education*, 19(1): 324. doi: https://doi.org/10.1186/s12909-019-1762-0

Gordon-Burns, D. & Walker, H.P. (2015). Institutionalised racism in the public health system. *New Zealand Journal of Occupational Therapy*, 62(2): 43–47. Available at: https://link.gale.com/apps/doc/A514565898/AONE?u=anon~319082bb&sid=googleScholar&xid=326fcf66 accessed 28 September 2021

Graham. D.W. (2019). *Stanford Encyclopedia of Philosophy – Heraclitus*. Stanford, CA: The Metaphysics Research Lab., Stanford University. Available at: https://plato.stanford.edu/entries/heraclitus accessed 13 December 2022

Gregory, A. (2021). *Third of BAME staff in NHS mental health services face racist abuse at work.* Available at: www.theguardian.com/world/2021/sep/09/third-of-bame-staff-in-nhs-mental-health-services-face-racist-abuse-at-work accessed 5 February 2022

Grenier, M.-L. (2020). Cultural competency and the reproduction of white supremacy in occupational therapy education. *Health Education Journal*, 79(6): 633–644. doi: https://doi.org/10.1177/0017896920902515

Grenier, M-L., Zafran, H. & Roy, L. (2020). Current landscape of teaching diversity in occupational therapy education: A scoping review. *American Journal of Occupational Therapy*, 74(6): 7406205100p1–7406205100p15. doi: https://doi.org/10.5014/ajot.2020.044214

Grosfoguel, R. (2011). Decolonizing post-colonial studies and paradigms of political-economy: Transmodernity, decolonial thinking, and global coloniality. *Transmodernity: Journal of Peripheral Cultural Production of the Luso-Hispanic World*, 1(1) [online]. doi: https://doi.org/10.5070/T411000004

Grosfoguel, R. (2016). What is racism? *Journal of World-Systems Research*, 22(1): 9–15. doi: https://doi.org/10.5195/jwsr.2016.609

Grullon, E., Hunnicutt, C., Morrison, M., Langford, O. & Whaley, M. (2018). A need for occupational justice: The impact of racial microaggression on occupations, wellness and health promotion. Occupation: A medium of inquiry for students, faculty and other practitioners. *Advocating for Health through Occupational Studies*, 3(1): article 4. Available at: https://nsuworks.nova.edu/occupation/vol3/iss1/4 accessed 10 January 2022

Guajardo, A., Kronenberg, F. & Ramugondo, E.L. (2015). Southern occupational therapies: Emerging identities, epistemologies and practices. *South African Journal of Occupational Therapy*, 45(1): 3–10. doi: https://doi.org/10.17159/2310-3833/2015/v45n1a2

Guajardo Córdoba, A. (2020). About new forms of colonization in occupational therapy. Reflections on the idea of occupational justice from a critical-political philosophy perspective. *Cadernos Brasileiros de Terapia Ocupacional*, 28(4). doi: https://doi.org/10.4322/2526-8910.ctoARF2175

Guillaumin, C. & O'Callaghan, M. (1980). *Sociological Theories: Race and Colonialism*. Geneva, Switzerland: UNESCO

Hagiwara, N., Kron, F.W., Scerbo, M.W. & Watson, G.S. (2020). A call for grounding implicit bias training in clinical and translational frameworks. *The Lancet*, 395(10234): 1457–1460. doi: https://doi.org/10.1016/S0140-6736(20)30846-1

Hahn, R.A., Truman, B.I. & Williams, D.R. (2018). Civil rights as determinants of public health and racial and ethnic health equity: Health care, education, employment, and housing in the United States. *Social Science and Medicine – Population Health*, 4: 17–24. doi: https://doi.org/10.1016/j.ssmph.2017.10.006

Hamer, K., McFarland, S., Czarnecka, B., Golińska, A. *et al.* (2020). What is an 'ethnic group' in ordinary people's eyes? Different ways of understanding it among American, British, Mexican, and Polish respondents. *Cross-Cultural Research*, 54(1): 28–72. doi: https://doi.org/10.1177/1069397118816939

Hammell, K.W. (2009). Sacred texts: A sceptical exploration of the assumptions underpinning theories of occupation. *Canadian Journal of Occupational Therapy*, 76(1): 6–22. doi: https://doi.org/10.1177%2F000841740907600105

Hammell, K.W. (2011). Resisting theoretical imperialism in the disciplines of occupational science and occupational therapy. *British Journal of Occupational Therapy*, 74(1): 27–33. doi: https://doi.org/10.4276/030802211X12947686093602

Hammell, K.W. (2013). Occupation, well-being, and culture: Theory and cultural humility. *Canadian Journal of Occupational Therapy*, 80(4): 224–234. doi: https://doi.org/10.1177/0008417413500465

Hammell, K.W. (2021). Occupation in natural environments: Health equity and environmental justice. *Canadian Journal of Occupational Therapy*, 88(4): 319–328. doi: https://doi.org/10.1177/00084174211040000

Hammer, M.R., Bennett, M.J. & Wiseman, R. (2003). The intercultural development inventory: A measure of intercultural sensitivity. *International Journal of Intercultural Relations*, 27(4): 421–443. doi: https://doi.org/10.1016/S0147-1767(03)00032-4

Hammond, J., Williams, A., Walker, S. & Norris, M. (2019). Working hard to belong: A qualitative study exploring students from black, Asian and minority ethnic backgrounds experiences of pre-registration physiotherapy education. *BMC Medical Education*, 19 (Article 372) [online]. doi: https://doi.org/10.1186/s12909-019-1821-6

Harro, B. (2000). The Cycle of Socialization. In M. Adams, W.J. Blumenfeld, R. Castañeda, H.W. Hackman, M.L. Peters & X. Zuniga (eds), *Readings for Diversity and Social Justice* (pp.16–21). London: Psychology Press

Health and Care Professions Council (HCPC). (2021). *Reflective Practice*. London: HCPC. Available at: www.hcpc-uk.org/standards/meeting-our-standards/reflective-practice accessed 8 January 2022

Health and Care Professions Council (HCPC). (2022). *Occupational Therapy Standards of Proficiency*. London: HCPC. Available at: www.hcpc-uk.org/standards/standards-of-proficiency/occupational-therapists accessed 10 November 2022

Hess-April, L.A., Smith, J. & De Jongh, J.C. (2016). Exploring occupational therapy graduates' conceptualisations of occupational justice in practice: Curriculum implications. *African Journal of Health Professions Education*, 8(2): 189–192. doi: https://doi.org/10.7196/AJHPE.2016.v8i2.609

Hewett, R., Liefooghe, A., Visockaite, G. & Roongrerngsuke, S. (2018). Bullying at work: Cognitive appraisal of negative act and the impact on wellbeing and performance. *Journal of Occupational Health Psychology*, 23(1): 71–84. doi: https://doi.org/10.1037/ocp0000064

Hills Collins, P. & Bilge, S. (2020). Intersectionality (second edition). Cambridge: Polity Press.

Hocking, C. (2017). Occupational justice and social justice: The moral claim for inclusion. *Journal of Occupational Science*, 24(1): 29–42. doi: https://doi.org/10.1080/14427591.2017.1294016

Hodge, K. & Marsh, S. (2015). Teaching profession fails to reflect multi-cultural student population. *The Guardian*. Available at: www.theguardian.com/teacher-network/2015/nov/19/teaching-fails-reflect-multi-cultural-student-population accessed 31 May 2021

Home Office. (2021). *Stop and Search*. Available at: www.ethnicity-facts-figures.service.gov.uk/crime-justice-and-the-law/policing/stop-and-search/latest accessed 19 February 2022

Hordge-Freeman, E. & Loblack, A. (2020). 'Cops only see the brown skin, they could care less where it originated': Afro-Latinx perceptions of the #BlackLivesMatter Movement. *Sociological Perspectives*, 64(4): 518–535. doi: https://doi.org/10.1177/0731121420961135

Howard University. (2018). *Black Lives Matter Movement*. Available at: https://library.law.howard.edu/civilrightshistory/BLM accessed 28 December 2021

Huff, S., Rudman, D.L., Magalhães, L., Lawson, E. & Kanyamala, M. (2020). Enacting a critical decolonizing ethnographic approach in occupation-based research. *Journal of Occupational Science*, 1–15. doi: https://doi.org/10.1080/14427591.2020.1824803

Ife, J. (2008). *Human Rights and Social Work. Towards Rights Based Practice*. Cambridge: Cambridge University Press

Ihollaback. (2021). Conflict De-Escalation: A how-to guide. *Hollaback! Together We Have the Power to End Harassment*. Available at: www.ihollaback.org/conflict-de-escalation-a-how-to-guide accessed 24 June 2022

Inoue, A.B. (2015). Chapter 5: Designing Antiracist Writing Assessment Ecologies. In *Antiracist Writing Assessment Ecologies: Teaching and Assessing Writing for a Socially Just Future* (pp.283–300). South Carolina: Parlor Press LLC

Iwama, M. (2003). Toward culturally relevant epistemologies in occupational therapy. *American Journal of Occupational Therapy*, 57(5): 582–588. doi: https://doi.org/10.5014/ajot.57.5.582

Iwama, M. (2004). Meaning and inclusion: Revising culture in occupational therapy. *The Australian Occupational Therapy Journal*, 51(1): 1–2. doi: https://doi.org/10.1111/j.1440-1630.2004.00429.x

Iwama, M. (2005). Situated Meaning: An Issue of Culture, Inclusion, and Occupational Therapy. In F. Kronenberg, S.S. Algado & N. Pollard (eds), *Occupational Therapy Without Borders* (pp.127–139). Edinburgh: Churchill Livingstone Elsevier

Iwama, M. (2006). *Culturally Relevant Occupational Therapy*. London: Churchill Livingstone Elsevier

Iwama, M. (2007). Culture and occupational therapy: Meeting the challenge of relevance in a global world. *Occupational Therapy International*, 4(4): 183–187. doi: https://doi.org/10.1002/oti.234

Jemal, A. (2017). Critical consciousness: A critique and critical analysis of the literature. *Urban Review November*, 49(4): 602–626. doi: https://doi.org/10.1007/s11256-017-0411-3

Jones, J. & Mosher, W.D. (2013). *Fathers' Involvement With Their Children: United States, 2006–2010* (No. 71; National Health Statistics Reports, p.22). US Department of Health and Human Services

Johnson, K.R. & Lavalley, R. (2021). From racialized think-pieces toward anti-racist praxis in our science, education, and practice. *Journal of Occupational Science*, 28(3): 404–409. doi: https://doi.org/10.1080/14427591.2020.1847598

Johnson, R., Browning, K. & DeClerk, L. (2021). Strategies to reduce bias and racism in nursing precepted clinical experiences. *Journal of Nursing Education*, 60(12): 697–702. doi: https://doi.org/10.3928/01484834-20211103-01

Jordan, A., Allsop, A.Z.A.S. & Collins, P.Y. (2021). Decriminalising being Black with mental illness. *The Lancet Psychiatry*, 8(1): 8–9. doi: https://doi.org/10.1016/S2215-0366(20)30519-8

Jungersen, K. (1992). Culture, theory and the practice of occupational therapy in New Zealand/Aotearoa. *American Journal of Occupational Therapy*, 46(8), 745–750. doi: https://doi.org/10.5014/ajot.46.8.745

Kantartzis, S. & Molineux, M. (2011). The influence of western society's construction of a healthy daily life on the conceptualisation of occupation. *Journal of Occupational Science*, 18(1): 62–80. doi: https://doi.org/10.1080/14427591.2011.566917

Kendi, I.X. (2017). *Stamped from the Beginning: The Definitive History of Racist Ideas in America.* First trade paperback edition. New York, NY: Nation Books

Kendi, I.X. (2019). *How to Be an Antiracist.* London: The Bodley Head

Kerin, Ú. (2020). Professional socialisation processes help facilitate the transition from student to qualified nurse. *Evidence-Based Nursing,* 23(2): 47. doi: https://doi.org/10.1136/ebnurs-2019-103078

Kerner Commission. (1968). *Report of the National Advisory Commission on Civil Disorders.* Washington, DC: Kerner Commission. Available at: https://belonging.berkeley.edu/sites/default/files/kerner_commission_full_report.pdf?file=1&force=1 accessed 18 June 2022

Keshet, Y. & Popper-Giveon, A. (2017). Neutrality in medicine and health professionals from ethnic minority groups: The case of Arab health professionals in Israel. *Social Science and Medicine,* Feb, 174: 35–42. doi: https://doi.org/10.1016/j.socscimed.2016.12.019

Kiepek, N. & Beagan, B. (2018). Substance use and professional identity. *Contemporary Drug Problems,* 45(1): 47–66. doi: https://doi.org/10.1177/0091450917748982

King, M.L. Jr. (1963). *Strength to Love.* New York, NY: Harper & Row

King's Fund. (2020). *A long way to go: Ethnic minority NHS staff share their stories.* Available at: https://features.kingsfund.org.uk/2020/07/ethnic-minority-nhs-staff-racism-discrimination/index.html accessed 5 January 2022

Kingsley, P. & Molineux, M. (2000). True to our philosophy? Sexual orientation and occupation. *British Journal of Occupational Therapy,* 63(5): 205–210. doi: https://doi.org/10.1177/030802260006300504

Kinsella, E.A. & Whiteford, G.E. (2009). Knowledge generation and utilisation in occupational therapy: Towards epistemic reflexivity. *Australian Occupational Therapy Journal,* 56(4): 249–258. doi: https://doi.org/10.1111/j.1440-1630.2007.00726.x

Kline, R. (2014). *The 'snowy white peaks' of the NHS: A survey of discrimination in governance and leadership and the potential impact on patient care in London and England.* London: Middlesex University. Available at: www.barnsleyhospital.nhs.uk/equalitydiversity/files/2012/01/Roger-Kline-article.pdf accessed 10 March 2023

Kline, R. (2020). After the speeches: What now for NHS staff race discrimination? *BMJ Leader.* Available at: https://blogs.bmj.com/bmjleader/2020/06/13/after-the-speeches-what-now-for-nhs-staff-race-discrimination-by-roger-kline accessed 30 July 2021

Krefting, L. (1992). Strategies for the development of occupational therapy in the Third World. *American Journal of Occupational Therapy,* 46(8): 758–761. doi: https://doi.org/10.5014/ajot.46.8.758

Krishnagiri, S., Hooper, B., Price, P., Taff, S.D. & Bilics, A. (2017). Explicit or hidden? Exploring how occupation is taught in occupational therapy curricula in the United States. *American Journal of Occupational Therapy,* 71(2): 7102230020p1–7102230020p9. doi: https://doi.org/10.5014/ajot.2017.024174

Kronenberg, F. (2020a). *Undoing colonial-OT (Coloniality): Occupational therapy cultivating a praxis of doing well together in Ghana* [Keynote address]. Occupational Therapy Association of Ghana Congress, Korlebu, Accra, Ghana

Kronenberg, F. (2020b). *Systemic racism in occupational therapy: Dealing with the skeleton in our closets.* OT Show Conference. Available at: www.youtube.com/watch?v=NwIcdG65e5k accessed 28 December 2021

Kronenberg, F. (2021a). Commentary on JOS Editorial Board's anti-racism pledge. *Journal of Occupational Science,* 27(3): 398–403. doi: https://doi.org/10.1080/14427591.2020.1827483

Kronenberg, F. (2021b). *Podcast Episode Dr Frank Kronenberg 'A different kind of cat'. OT – What's your focus?* Interview by Farrah Money. Available at: https://open.spotify.com/episode/47B3rcEfLlu8s8ZqBWoTy6 accessed 7 March 2021

Kronenberg, F., Kathard, H., Rudman, D. & Ramugondo, E. (2015). Can post-apartheid South Africa be enabled to humanise and heal itself? *South African Journal of Occupational Therapy,* 45(1): 20–27. doi: http://dx.doi.org/10.17159/2310-3833/2015/v45n01a4

Kumagai, A.K. & Lypson, M.L. (2009). Beyond cultural competence: Critical consciousness, social justice, and multicultural education. *Academic Medicine,* 84(6): 782–787. doi: https://doi.org/10.1097/ACM.0b013e3181a42398

References

Kupperman, J.J. (2001). *Classic Asian Philosophy.* Oxford: Oxford University Press

Ladson-Billings, G. (1998). Just what is critical race theory and what's it doing in a nice field like education? *International Journal of Qualitative Studies in Education,* 11(1): 7–24. doi: https://doi.org/10.1080/095183998236863

Laing, A.F. (2021). Decolonising pedagogies in undergraduate geography: Student perspectives on a decolonial movements module. *Journal of Geography in Higher Education,* 45(1): 1–19. doi: https://doi.org/10.1080/03098265.2020.1815180

Laliberte Rudman, D. (2013). Enacting the critical potential of occupational science: Problematizing the individualizing of occupation. *Journal of Occupational Science,* 20(4): 298–313. doi: https://doi.org/10.1080/14427591.2013.803434

Laliberte Rudman, D. (2014). Embracing and enacting an 'occupational imagination': Occupational science as transformative. *Journal of Occupational Science,* 21(4): 373–388. doi: https://doi.org/10.1080/14427591.2014.888970

Laliberte-Rudman, D., Dennhardt, S., Fok, D., Huot, S. *et al.* (2008). A vision for occupational science: Reflecting on our disciplinary culture. *Journal of Occupational Science,* 15(3): 136–146. doi: https://doi.org/10.1080/14427591.2008.9686623

Lammy, D. (2017). *The Lammy Review: An Independent Review into the Treatment of, and Outcomes for, Black, Asian and Minority Ethnic Individuals in the Criminal Justice System.* London, HM Inspectorate of Probation, The Work of Probation Services in Courts

Lamont, A. (2021). *Guide to Allyship.* Amélie Studio. Available at: https://guidetoallyship.com accessed 24 June 2022

The Lancet (2022). The Lancet Series on racism, xenophobia, discrimination, and health. Available at: www.thelancet.com/series/racism-xenophobia-discrimination-health accessed 11 June 2022

Lang, B. (2000). *Race and Racism in Theory and Practice.* Washington, DC: Rowman & Littlefield

Lavalley, R. & Robinson Johnson, K. (2022). Occupation, injustice, and anti-Black racism in the United States of America. *Journal of Occupational Science,* 29(4): 487–499. doi: https://doi.org/10.1080/14427591.2020.1810111

Leite Junior, J.D., Farias, M.N. & Martins, S. (2021). Dona Ivone Lara and Occupational Therapy: The becoming-black of the profession's history. *Brazilian Journal of Occupational Therapy,* 29. doi: https://doi.org/10.1590/2526-8910.ctoarf2171

Limb, M. (2021). Disparity in maternal deaths because of ethnicity is 'unacceptable'. *BMJ,* 372: n152. doi: https://doi.org/10.1136/bmj.n152

Liyanage, M. (2020). *Miseducation: Decolonising Curricula, Culture and Pedagogy in UK Universities, Debate Paper 23.* Oxford: Higher Education Policy Institute

Lock, M., Williams, M., Lloyd-Haynes, A., Burmeiter, O. *et al.* (2021). Are cultural safety definitions culturally safe? A review of 42 cultural safety definitions in an Australian cultural concept soup [pre-print]. doi: https://doi.org/10.21203/rs.3.rs-1179330/v1. Available at: www.academia.edu/66462745/Are_cultural_safety_definitions_culturally_safe_A_review_of_42_cultural_safety_definitions_in_an_Australian_cultural_concept_soup accessed 21 September 2022

Lopes, R.E. & Malfitano, A.P.S. (2020). *Social Occupational Therapy: Theoretical and Practical Designs.* Phildephia, PA: Elsevier

Lopez-Littleton, V., Blessett, B. & Burr, J. (2018). Advancing social justice and racial equity in the public sector. *Journal of Public Affairs Education,* 24(4), 449–468

Lorde, A. (1994). The Master's Tools Will Never Dismantle the Master's House. In *Sister Outsider: Essays and Speeches* (pp.110–114). Berkeley, CA: Crossing Press. [print 2007]. Available at: https://collectiveliberation.org/wp-content/uploads/2013/01/Lorde_The_Masters_Tools.pdf accessed 24 June 2022

Lucas, C. & Washington, S. (2020). *Understanding Systemic Racism in the United States: Educating Our Students and Ourselves.* USA: American Occupational Therapy Association Continuing Education Article CEA1020

Mackenbach, J.P. & Bakker, M.J. (2003). Tackling socioeconomic inequalities in health: Analysis of European experiences. *The Lancet,* 362(9393): 1409–1414. doi: https://doi.org/10.1016/S0140-6736(03)14639-9

Mahoney, W.J. & Kiraly-Alvarez, A.F. (2019). Challenging the status quo: Infusing non-Western ideas into occupational therapy education and practice. *The Open Journal of Occupational Therapy*, 7(3): 1–10. doi: https://doi.org/10.15453/2168-6408.1592

Malfitano, A.P.S., Cruz, D.M.C. & Lopes, R.E. (2020). Occupational therapy in times of pandemic: Social security and guaranties of possible everyday life for all. *Cadernos Brasileira de Terapia Ocupacional*, 28(2): 401–404. doi: https://doi.org/10.4322/2526-8910.ctoED22802

Malfitano, A.P.S., Lopes, R.E., Magalhães, L. & Townsend, E.A. (2014). Social occupational therapy: Conversations about a Brazilian experience. *Canadian Journal of Occupational Therapy*, 81(5): 298–307. doi: https://doi.org/10.1177/0008417414536712

Malfitano, A.P.S., Pan, L. & Sousa, A. (2022). *Presentation for DisruptOT 30th April Social Occupational Therapy Youth, Communities and Public School*. Bay Area, CA: DisruptOT

Malkawi, S.H., Alqatarneh, N.S. & Fehringer, E.K. (2020). The influence of culture on occupational therapy practice in Jordan. *Occupational Therapy International* [online], 1092805: 1–9. doi: https://doi.org/10.1155/2020/1092805

Mandela, N. (2011). *Nelson Mandela By Himself: The Authorised Book of Quotations*. Johannesburg: Pan Macmillan

Maphumulo, W. & Bhengu, B. (2019). Challenges of quality improvement in the healthcare of South Africa post-apartheid: A critical review. *Curationis*, 42(1): 1–9. doi: https://doi.org/10.4102/curationis.v42i1.1901

Marder, A. (2017). *7 studies that prove the value of diversity in the work place*. Arlington, VA: Capterra. Available at: https://blog.capterra.com/7-studies-that-prove-the-value-of-diversity-in-the-workplace accessed 15 March 2021

Mariotti, M. & Fourie, J. (2014). The economics of apartheid: An introduction. *History of Developing Regions*, 29(2): 113–125. doi: https://doi.org/10.1080/20780389.2014.958298

Marmot, M. (2010). *Fair Society, Health Lives: Marmot Review, Strategic Review of Health Inequalities in post 2010*. London: The Marmot Review

Marmot, M., Allen, J., Boyce, T., Goldblatt, P. & Morrison, J. (2020a). *Health Equity in England: The Marmot Review 10 years on*. London: Institute of Health Equity. Available at: www.health.org.uk/publications/reports/the-marmot-review-10-years-on accessed 28 December 2022

Marmot, M., Allen, J., Goldblatt, P., Herd, E. & Morrison, J. (2020b). *'Build Back Fairer': The COVID-19 Marmot Review. The Pandemic, Socioeconomic and Health Inequalities in England*. London: The Health Foundation and Institute of Health Equity

Marmot, M. & Wilkinson, R.G. (2005). *Social Determinants of Health*. Oxford: Oxford University Press

Martins, S. (2021). *Repercussões da experiência de racismo nas ocupações maternais de mulheres negras: estratégias de enfrentamento* [PhD thesis]. Federal University of São Carlos, São Carlos

Martins, S. & Farias, M.N. (2020). Práticas de terapia ocupacional e contexto sociocultural: caso de uma menina negra. In L.C.C. Gradim, T.N. Finarde & D.C.M. Carrijo (eds), *Práticas em Terapia Ocupacional* (pp.32–37). Barueri, Sao Paulo, Brazil: Editora Manole

Matebeni, D. (2012). Managing diversity in the workplace. *Nursing Update* (DENOSA) July, 37(7): 28

Matias, C.M. & Boucher, C. (2021). From critical whiteness studies to a critical study of whiteness: Restoring criticality in critical whiteness studies [online]. *Whiteness and Education*. doi: https://doi.org/10.1080/23793406.2021.1993751

Matsuda, M.J., Lawrence, C.R., Delgado, R. & Crenshaw, K.W. (1993). *Words that Wound: Critical Race Theory, Assaultive Speech, and the First Amendment*. Boulder, CO: Westview Press

McConnell, C. (2022). Racially informed care: A treatment approach and exploration of the implications of race related barriers in the United States. *The Open Journal of Occupational Therapy*, 10(1): 1–8 [Article 15]. doi: https://doi.org/10.15453/2168-6408.1888

McGregor-Smith, R. (2017). *Race in the workplace: The McGregor-Smith Review*. London: Crown Services Available at: https://assets.publishing.service.gov.uk/government/uploads/system/uploads/attachment_data/file/594336/race-in-workplace-mcgregor-smith-review.pdf accessed 10 January 2022

References

McLean, I. & McMillan, A. (2009). *The Concise Oxford Dictionary of Politics – Apartheid*. Oxford: Oxford University Press. Available at: www.oxfordreference.com/view/10.1093/acref/9780199207800.001.0001/acref-9780199207800-e-53 accessed 1 March 2022

McIntosh, P. (1989). White privilege: Unpacking the invisible knapsack. *Peace and Freedom Magazine*, July/August, pp.10–12. Available at: https://psychology.umbc.edu/wp-content/uploads/sites/57/2016/10/White-Privilege_McIntosh-1989.pdf accessed 22 June 2022

Melese, S. & Tadege, A. (2019). The Ethiopian curriculum development and implementation vis-à-vis Schwab's signs of crisis in the field of curriculum [online]. *Cogent Education*, 6(1). doi: https://doi.org/10.1080/2331186X.2019.1633147

Menakem, R. (n.d.). *Somatic abolitionism – Antiracist practices*. Available at: www.resmaa.com/movement accessed 23 June 2022

Menakem, R. (2022). *White Bodies and the Energies of Race: How our bodies can develop collective containers to handle the charge of race*. Available at: www.psychologytoday.com/us/blog/somatic-abolitionism/202203/white-bodies-and-the-energies-race accessed 23 June 2022

Meyer, O.L. & Zane, N. (2013). The influence of race and ethnicity in clients' experience of mental health treatment. *Journal of Community Psychology*, 41(7): 884–901. doi: https://doi.org/10.1002/jcop.21580

Miller, E.F. (1980). What does 'political' mean? *The Review of Politics*, Jan, 42(1): 56–72. doi: https://doi.org/10.1017/S0034670500030783

Milner, H.R. IV (2006). The Promise of Black Teachers' Success with Black Students. *Education Foundations*, 20(Summer-Fall): 89–104. Available at: https://files.eric.ed.gov/fulltext/EJ794734.pdf accessed 28 September 2021

Mind. (2020). *The mental health emergency: how has the coronavirus pandemic impacted our mental health?* London: Mind. Available at: www.mind.org.uk accessed 15 October 2021

Moorley, C., Darbyshire, P., Serrant, L., Mohamed, J., Ali, P. & De Souza, R. (2020). Dismantling structural racism: Nursing must not be caught on the wrong side of history. *Journal of Advanced Nursing*, 76(10): 2450–2453. doi: https://doi.org/10.1111/jan.14469

Muir, H. (2020). Cornel West: 'George Floyd's public lynching pulled the cover off who we really are'. *The Guardian*. Available at: www.theguardian.com/us-news/2020/oct/19/cornel-west-george-floyds-public-lynching-pulled-the-cover-off-who-we-really-are accessed 31 December 2021

Munanga, K. & Gomes, N.L. (2016). *O negro no Brasil de hoje* (second edition). Hershey, PA: Global

Muñoz, J.P. (2007). Culturally responsive caring in occupational therapy. *Occupational Therapy International*, 14(4): 256–280. doi: https://doi.org/10.1002/oti.238

Myers, E. (2017). *Beyond the Wages of Whiteness: Du Bois on the Irrationality of Antiblack Racism*. Available at: https://items.ssrc.org/reading-racial-conflict/beyond-the-wages-of-whiteness-du-bois-on-the-irrationality-of-antiblack-racism accessed 29 November 2021

National Association for the Advancement of Colored People (NAACP). (2022). *History of lynching in America*. Available at: https://naacp.org/find-resources/history-explained/history-lynching-america accessed 15 October 2022

National Institutes of Health. (2021). *Cultural Respect*. Bethesda, MD: National Institutes of Health. Available at: www.nih.gov/institutes-nih/nih-office-director/office-communications-public-liaison/clear-communication/cultural-respect accessed 23 June 2022

National Perinatal Epidemiology Unit and University of Oxford. (2021). *MBRRACE-UK Saving Lives, Improving Mothers' Care Lay Summary Report*. Available at: www.npeu.ox.ac.uk/assets/downloads/mbrrace-uk/reports/maternal-report-2021/MBRRACE-UK_Maternal_Report_2021_-_Lay_Summary_v10.pdf accessed 2 January 2022

Ndaa, P. (2014). Professional Occupational Therapy in Ghana: Taking the Initiative in the Sub-Region. In S. Antwi-Bafour, B. Ajideran, P. Ayeh-kumi, S. Anim Sampong *et al.* (eds), *Contributions of Allied Health Science to Healthcare Delivery in Ghana* (pp.112–126). University of Ghana: Digibooks Ghana Ltd

Ndlovu-Gatsheni, S.J. (2015). Decoloniality as the future of Africa. *History Compass*, 13(10): 485–496. doi: https://doi.org/10.1111/hic3.12264

Ndlovu-Gatsheni, S. (2020). *Decolonization, Decoloniality, and the Future of African Studies: A Conversation with Dr. Sabelo Ndlovu-Gatsheni*. Available at: https://items.ssrc.org/from-our-programs/decolonization-decoloniality-and-the-future-of-african-studies-a-con-versation-with-dr-sabelo-ndlovu-gatsheni accessed 16 November 2021

Nelson, A. (2007). Seeing white: A critical exploration of occupational therapy with Indige-nous Australian people. *Occupational Therapy International*, 14(4): 327–255. doi: https://doi.org/10.1002/oti.236

Newman, D.M. (2012). *Sociology: Exploring the Architecture of Everyday Life* (ninth edition). Los Angeles, CA: Sage

NHS Digital. (2022). *Detentions Under the Mental Health Act – GOV.UK Ethnicity Facts and Figures*. Available at: www.ethnicity-facts-figures.service.gov.uk/health/mental-health/detentions-under-the-mental-health-act/latest accessed 15 October 2022

NHS England. (2020). *Menu of Evidence-Based Interventions and Approaches for Addressing and Reducing Health Inequalities*. Available at: https://webarchive.nationalarchives.gov.uk/ukgwa/20211101142354/https:/www.england.nhs.uk/ltphimenu accessed 28 December 2021

NHS England. (2021). *Workforce Race Equality Standards Data 2020*. Available at: www.eng-land.nhs.uk/wp-content/uploads/2021/02/Workforce-Race-Equality-Standard-2020-re-port.pdf accessed 28 December 2021

Nicholls, L. & Elliot, M.L. (2019). In the shadow of occupation: Racism, shame and grief. *Journal of Occupational Science*, 26(3): 354–365. doi: https://doi.org/10.1080/14427591.2018.1523021

Nkosi, B. & Daniels, P. (2007). Family strengths. *Marriage & Family Review*, 41(1–2): 11–26. doi: https://doi.org/10.1300/J002v41n01_02

Noman, N. (2020). *'Blackout Tuesday' on Instagram was a teachable moment for allies like me*. THINK: Opinion, Analysis, Essays. Available at: www.nbcnews.com/think/opinion/blackout-tuesday-instagram-was-teachable-moment-allies-me-ncna1225961 accessed 24 June 2022

Obama, M. (2011). *Remarks by The First Lady during Keynote Address at Young African Women Leaders Forum*. Available at: https://obamawhitehouse.archives.gov/the-press-of-fice/2011/06/22/remarks-first-lady-during-keynote-address-young-african-women-leaders-fo accessed 10 February 2023

Occupational Therapy Association of South Africa (OTASA). (2018). *Short History of OTASA – How it all began*. Available at: https://otasa.org.za/about-us/history accessed 24 May 2021

Occupational Therapy Magazine. (2020). *Open letter to RCOT regarding their diversity state-ment*. Available at: https://ot-magazine.co.uk/open-letter-to-rcot-regarding-their-di-versity-statement accessed 29 March 2021

Oliver, D. (2021). Wider health determinants aren't just for pandemics. *BMJ*, 372: n276. doi: https://doi.org/10.1136/bmj.n276. Available at: www.bmj.com/content/372/bmj.n276 accessed 10 June 2021

Oluo, I. (2017). *So You Want to Talk About Race*. Seattle, WA: Seal Press

Ontario Human Rights Commission. (2018). *Interrupted childhoods: Over-representation of Indigenous and Black children in Ontario child welfare*. Available at: www.ohrc.on.ca/en/interrupted-childhoods accessed 22 June 2022

Opoku, E.N., Van Niekerk, L. & Khuabi, L.A.J.N. (2022). Exploring the transition from student to health professional by the first cohort of locally trained occupational therapists in Ghana. *Scandinavian Journal of Occupational Therapy*, 29(1): 46–57. doi: https://doi.org/10.1080/11038128.2020.1865448

Owens, L. (2016). Our Professional Existence Is Political: Critical Reflections on Seeing 'White' in the Profession. In D. Sakellariou & N. Pollard (eds), *Occupational Therapies Without Borders E-Book: Integrating Justice With Practice* (pp.194–202). Amsterdam, Holland: Elsevier Health Sciences

Palmer, R.T. & Maramba, D.C. (2015). Racial microaggressions among Asian American and Latino/a students at a historically black university. *Journal of College Student Develop-ment*, 56(7): 705–722. doi: https://doi.org/10.1353/csd.2015.0076

References

Parker, R. & Badger, J. (2018). *The Essential Guide for Newly Qualified Occupational Therapists – Transition to Practice*. London: Jessica Kingsley Publishers

PBS. (1993). *Toni Morrison Interview with Charlie Rose* [video]. Available at: https://charlierose. com/videos/18778 accessed 9 July 2022

Pentland, D. & Pentland, B. (2015). Sir David K Henderson and the origins of British occupational therapy. *Scottish Medical Journal*, 60(4): 249–251. doi: https://doi. org/10.1177/0036933015596143

Perera, I. & Douglas, K.-L. (2020). *A Here-And-Now Challenge for Occupational Therapists*. Available at: https://rehab.queensu.ca/blog/here-and-now-challenge-occupation-al-therapists accessed 10 January 2022

Perryman-Fox, M. & Cox, D.L. (2020). Occupational therapy in the United Kingdom: Past, present, and future. *Annals of International Occupational Therapy*, 3(3): 144–151. doi: https://doi.org/10.3928/24761222-20200309-03

Phenix, A. & Grenier, M.-L. (2020). Shifting the ethical stance: Decolonising OT education [Class Lecture McGill University, Faculty of Physical and Occupational Therapy]

Picower, B. (2009). The unexamined Whiteness of teaching: How White teachers maintain and enact dominant racial ideologies. *Race, Ethnicity and Education*, 12(2): 197–215. doi: https://doi.org/10.1080/13613320902995475

Pilkington, E. (2021). 'Truth-telling has to happen': the museum of America's racist history. *The Guardian*. Available at: www.theguardian.com/us-news/2021/sep/19/the-legacy-mu-seum-america-racist-history accessed 16 June 2021

Pirbhai-Illich, F., Pete, S. & Martin, F. (2017). *Culturally Responsive Pedagogy: Working Towards Decolonization, Indigeneity, and Interculturalism*. Switzerland: Springer International Publishing

Pollard, N., & Sakellariou, D. (2012). The Language of Occupation. In N. Pollard & D. Sakellar-iou (eds), *Politics of Occupation-Centred Practice: Reflections on Occupational Engagement Across Cultures* (pp.25–41). Oxford: John Wiley and Sons

Pollard, N., & Sakellariou, D. (2014). The occupational therapist as a political being. *Cadernos de Terapia Ocupacional Da UFSCar*, 22(3), 643–652. doi: https://doi.org/10.4322/cto.2014.087

Pollard, N. Sakellariou, D. & Kronenberg, F. (2009). *Political Practice in Occupational Therapy*. London: Churchill Livingstone

Proctor, S.L., Kyle, J., Lau, C., Fefer, K. & Fischetti, J. (2016). Racial microaggressions and school psychology students: Who gets targeted and how intern supervisors can facilitate racial justice. *School Psychology Forum*, Fall, 10(3): 321–336

Public Health England. (2020a). *Beyond the Data: Understanding the Impact of COVID-19 on BAME Groups*. Available at: https://assets.publishing.service.gov.uk/government/uploads/system/uploads/attachment_data/file/892376/COVID_stakeholder_engage-ment_synthesis_beyond_the_data.pdf accessed 15 October 2020

Public Health England. (2020b). *Disparities in the Risk and Outcomes of COVID-19*. London: PHE Publications. Available at: https://assets.publishing.service.gov.uk/government/uploads/system/uploads/attachment_data/file/908434/Disparities_in_the_risk_and_outcomes_of_COVID_August_2020_update.pdf accessed 14 December 2021

Public Health England. (2020c). *Protecting and Improving the Nation's Health – Beyond the Data: Understanding the Impact of COVID-19 on BAME Groups*. London: PHE Publications

Quijano, A (2000). Coloniality of power, Eurocentrism and Latin America. *Nepantla: Views from the South*, 1(3): 533–580. Available at: https://edisciplinas.usp.br/pluginfile. php/347342/mod_resource/content/1/Quijano%20(2000)%20Colinality%20of%20power. pdf accessed 12 December 2021

Rammohan, I. (2019). *Why do Indigenous people in Canada face worse health outcomes than non-Indigenous people?* Available at: https://thevarsity.ca/2019/09/15/why-do-canadas-indigenous-people-face-worse-health-outcomes-than-non-indigenous-people accessed 19 July 2021

Ramugondo, E. (2000). *The Experience of Being an Occupational Therapy Student with an Underrepresented Ethnic and Cultural Background* [MA thesis]. Available at: https://open. uct.ac.za/handle/11427/3455 accessed 28 April 2021

Ramugondo, E.L. (2015). Occupational consciousness. *Journal of Occupational Science*, 22(4), 488–501. doi: https://doi.org/10.1080/14427591.2015.1042516

Ramugondo, E.L. (2018). Healing work: Intersections for decoloniality. *World Federation of Occupational Therapists Bulletin*, 74(2), 83–91. doi: https://doi.org/10.1080/1447382 8.2018.1523981

Ramugondo, E.L. (2020). *Whose lives matter in the Academy*. HELTASA Conference. Available at: https://m.youtube.com/watch?v=ng4QeWtv78w&feature=youtu.be accessed 31 December 2021

Ramugondo, E.L. & Kronenberg, F. (2015). Explaining collective occupations from a human relations perspective: Building the individual-collective dichotomy. *Journal of Occupational Science*, 22(11): 3–16. doi: https://doi.org/10.1080/14427591.2013.781920

Rangachari, P. & Woods, J. L. (2020). Preserving organizational resilience, patient safety, and staff retention during COVID-19 requires a holistic consideration of the psychological safety of healthcare workers. *International Journal of Environmental Research and Public Health*, 17(12): 4267. doi: https://doi.org/10.3390/ijerph17124267

Razack, S. (1995). The perils of talking about culture: Schooling research on South and East Asian students. *Race, Gender and Class*, 2(3): 67–82. Available at: www.jstor.org/stable/41674709 accessed 15 June 2022

Razai, M.S., Kankam, H.K. N., Majeed, A., Esmail, A. & Williams, D.R. (2021). Mitigating ethnic disparities in COVID-19 and beyond. *BMJ*, 372: m4921. doi: https://doi.org/10.1136/bmj.m4921. Available at: www.bmj.com/content/bmj/372/bmj.m4921.full.pdf accessed 10 March 2023

Reza, J.N. & van Heel, D. (2022). *Diabetes and Heart Disease in Bangladeshis and Pakistanis*. London: Queen Mary's University London. Available at: www.genesandhealth.org/genes-your-health/diabetes-and-heart-disease-bangladeshis-and-pakistanis accessed 23 June 2022

Ribeiro, R.P. (2021). *Uma cartografia bibliográfica da terapia ocupacional social sobre a temática da juventude negra* [MA thesis]. Federal University of Espirito Santo

Richards, L.-A. & Galvaan, R. (2018). Developing a socially transformative focus in Occupational Therapy: insights from South African practice. *South African Journal of Occupational Therapy*, 48(1): 3–8. doi: https://doi.org/10.17159/2310-3833/2017/vol48n1a2

Ridgeway, M.L. & McGee, E.O. (2018). Black mathematics educators: Researching toward racial emancipation of black students. *The Urban Review*, 50(2): 301–322. doi: https://doi.org/10.1007/s11256-018-0452-2

Rittel, H.W.J. & Webber, M.M. (1973). Dilemmas in a general theory of planning. *Policy Sciences*, 4: 155–169. doi: https://doi.org/10.1007/BF01405730

Rock, D. & Grant, H. (2016). *Why diverse teams are smarter*. Boston, MA: Harvard Business Review. Available at: https://hbr.org/2016/11/why-diverse-teams-are-smarter accessed 21 June 2022

Rock, D., Grant, H. & Grey, J. (2016). *Diverse teams feel less comfortable and that's why they perform better*. Boston, MA: Harvard Business Review. Available at: https://hbr.org/2016/09/diverse-teams-feel-less-comfortable-and-thats-why-they-perform-better accessed 29 June 2022

Rojas, F. (2020). Moving beyond the rhetoric: A comment on Szetela's critique of the Black Lives Matter movement. *Ethnic and Racial Studies*, 43(8): 1407–1413. doi: https://doi.org/10.1080/01419870.2020.1718725

Roots of Justice. (2014). *Building an Effective White Caucus*. Available at: www.rootsofjustice-training.org/uploads/1/3/9/1/139148852/white-caucus-faq.pdf accessed 10 February 2023

Royal College of Occupational Therapists (RCOT). (2021a). *What is occupational therapy?* Available at: www.rcot.co.uk/about-occupational-therapy/what-is-occupational-therapy accessed 22 December 2021

Royal College of Occupational Therapists (RCOT). (2021b). *Professional standards for occupational therapy practice, conduct and ethics*. Available at: www.rcot.co.uk/publications/professional-standards-occupational-therapy-practice-conduct-and-ethics accessed 10 January 2022

References

Rudman, D., Pollard, N., Craig, C., Kantartzis, S. *et al.* (2018). Contributing to social transformation through occupation: Experiences from a Think Tank. *Journal of Occupational Science*, 26(2): 1–7. doi: https://doi.org/10.1080/14427591.2018.1538898

Rutherford, A. (2020). *How to Argue with a Racist*. London: Wiedenfield & Nicholson

Ryan, A., Gilroy, J. & Gibson, C. (2020). #Changethedate: Advocacy as an on-line and decolonising occupation. *Journal of Occupational Science*, 27(3): 405–416. doi: https://doi.org/10.1080/14427591.2020.1759448

Sacks, V. & Murphey, D. (2018). *The prevalence of adverse childhood experiences, nationally, by state, and by race or ethnicity*. Available at: www.childtrends.org/publications/prevalence-adverse-childhood-experiences-nationally-state-race-ethnicity accessed 16 June 2022

Said, E.W. (1993). *Culture and Imperialism*. New York, NY: Vintage

Saini, A. (2019). *Superior: The Return of Race Science*. London: 4th Estate

Sakellariou, D. & Pollard, N. (2012). Narratives and Truths. In N. Pollard & D. Sakellariou (eds), *Politics of Occupation-Centred Practice: Reflections on Occupational Engagement Across Cultures* (pp.81–91). Oxford: John Wiley and Sons

Sakellariou, D. & Pollard, N. (2013). A commentary on the social responsibility of occupational therapy. *Journal of Further and Higher Education*, 37(3): 416–430. doi: https://doi.org/10.1080/0309877X.2011.645459

Sakellariou, D. & Pollard, N. (eds). (2017). *Occupational Therapies without Borders: Integrating Justice with Practice*. Edinburgh: Elsevier

Salvan, L. (2013). Cultural responsibility. Small steps to restore anthropology in economic behaviour. Interviews and best practices. *Tafter Journal*, September, 63. Available at: www.tafterjournal.it/2013/09/09/cultural-responsibility-small-steps-to-restore-anthropology-in-economic-behaviour-interviews-and-best-practices accessed 8 January 2021

Samson, S. (2018). *Class-action lawyer told of 2 coerced sterilizations of Indigenous women in Manitoba*. CBC News, 14 November. Available at: www.cbc.ca/news/canada/manitoba/manitoba indigenous-women-forced-sterilization-lawsuit-1.4904421 accessed 29 June 2022

Santos, I.A.A. (2013). *Direitos humanos e as práticas de racismo*. Câmara dos Deputados, Edições Câmara, Brasília, Distrito Federal – Brazil

Santos, M.P.A., Nery, J.S., Goes, E.F., DaSilva, A. *et al.* (2020). População negra e COVID-19: reflexões sobre racismo e saúde. *Estudos Avançados*, 34(99): 225–244. doi: https://doi.org/10.1590/s0103-4014.2020.3499.014

Sarfo-Annin, J.K. (2020). Ethnic inclusion in medicine: The ineffectiveness of the 'Black, Asian and Minority Ethnic' metric to measure progress. *BJGP Open*, 4(5). doi: https://doi.org/10.3399/bjgpo.2020.0155

Schaefer, R.T. (ed.). (2008). *Encyclopedia of Race, Ethnicity, and Society*. Thousand Oaks, CA: Sage Publications

Scharmer, O. (2015). *Otto Scharmer on the 4 levels of listening*. Available at: www.youtube.com/watch?v=eLfXpRkVZaI accessed 10 January 2022

Scherff, L. & Spector, K. (eds). (2011). *Culture, Relevance, and Schooling: Exploring Uncommon Ground*. Lanham, MD: Rowman and Littlefield

Schouler-Ocak, M., Graef-Calliess, I.T., Tarricone, I., Qureshi, A., Katrup, M.C. & Bhugra, D. (2015). EPA guidance on cultural competence training. *European Psychiatry*, 30(3): 431–440. doi: https://doi.org/10.1016/j.eurpsy.2015.01.012

Sekulić, D. (2008). Ethnic Group. In R.T. Schaefer (ed.), *Encyclopedia of Race, Ethnicity, and Society* (pp.456–459). Thousand Oaks, CA: Sage Publications

Sensoy, Ö. & DiAngelo, R. (2017). 'We are all for diversity, but...': How faculty hiring committees reproduce whiteness and practical suggestions for how they can change. *Harvard Educational Review*, 87(4): 557–580. doi: https://doi.org/10.17763/1943-5045-87.4.557

Shirley, D. (2016). How to lead educational change. *Journal of Educational Change*, 17(3): 281–228. doi: https://doi.org/10.1007/s10833-016-9281-9

Simaan, J. (2017). Olive growing in Palestine: A decolonial ethnographic study of collective daily-forms-of-resistance. *Journal of Occupational Science*, 24(4): 510–523. doi: https://doi.org/10.1080/14427591.2017.1378119

Simaan, J. (2020a). Decolonising the curriculum is an ongoing and collective effort: Responding to Townsend (2020) and Gibson and Farias (2020). *Journal of Occupational Science*, 27(4): 563–568. doi: https://doi.org/10.1080/14427591.2020.1827696

Simaan, J. (2020b). Decolonising occupational science education through learning activities based on a study from the Global South. *Journal of Occupational Science*, 27(3): 432–442. doi: https://doi.org/10.1080/14427591.2020.1780937

Simó Algado, S., Córdoba, A.G., Oliver, F.C., Galheigo, S.M. & García-Ruiz, S. (eds). (2016). *Terapias ocupacionales desde el sur* (first edition). Santiago, Chile: Editorial Universidad de Santiago de Chile

Smedley, A. (1998). 'Race' and the construction of human identity. *American Anthropologist*, 100(3): 690–702. doi: https://doi.org/10.1525/aa.1998.100.3.690

Smedley, B.D. (2012). The lived experience of race and its health consequences. *American Journal of Public Health*, 102(5): 933–935. doi: https://doi.org/10.2105/AJPH.2011.300643

Smedley, B.D., Stith, A.Y. & Nelson, A.R. (2003). *Unequal Treatment: Confronting Racial and Ethnic Disparities in Health Care – Institute of Medicine (US) Committee on Understanding and Eliminating Racial and Ethnic Disparities in Health Care*. Washington, DC: National Academies Press (US)

Smiley, C.J. & Fakunle, D. (2016). From 'brute' to 'thug:' The demonization and criminalization of unarmed Black male victims. *American Journal of Human Behaviour in the Social Environment*, 26(3–4): 350–366. doi: https://doi.org/10.1080/10911359.2015.1129256

Smith, M.D. (2017). The dangerous myth of the 'missing black father.' *Washington Post*. Available at: www.washingtonpost.com/posteverything/wp/2017/01/10/the-dangerous-myth-of-the-missing-black-father accessed 15 June 2022

Smith, L. (2010). *Psychology, Poverty and the End of Social Exclusion: Putting Our Practice to Work*. New York, NY: Columbia University

Solorzano, D.G. & Yosso, T.J. (2001). Critical race and LatCrit theory and method: Counter-storytelling. *International Journal of Qualitative Studies in Education*, 14(4): 471–495. doi: https://doi.org/10.1080/09518390110063365

Spiliotopoulou, G. (2007). Preparing occupational therapy students for practice placements: Initial evidence. *British Journal of Occupational Therapy*, 70(9): 384–388. doi: https://doi.org/10.1177/030802260707000903

Stanley, J., Harris, R., Cormack, D., Waa, A. & Edwards, R. (2019). The impact of racism on the future health of adults: Protocol for a prospective cohort study. *BMC Public Health*, 19(346). doi: https://doi.org/10.1186/s12889-019-6664-x

Sterman, J. & Njelesani, J. (2021). Becoming anti-racist occupational therapy practitioners: A scoping study. *OTJR: Occupation, Participation and Health*, 41(4): 232–242. doi: https://doi.org/10.1177/15394492211019931

Stubbs, A. (ed.). (1978). *Steve Biko – I Write What I Like*. London: Bowerdean Press

Sue, D.W., Alsaidi, S., Awad, M.N., Glaeser, E., Calle, C.Z. & Mendez, N. (2019). Disarming racial microaggressions: Microintervention strategies for targets, White allies, and bystanders. *American Psychologist*, 74(1): 128–142. doi: https://doi.org/10.1037/amp0000296

Sue, D.W., Capodilupo, C.M., Torino, G.C., Bucceri, J.M. *et al.* (2007a). Racial microaggressions in everyday life: Implications for clinical practice. *American Psychologist*, 62(4): 271–286. doi: https://doi.org/10.1037/0003-066X.62.4.271

Sue, D.W., Nadal, K.L., Capodilupo, C.M., Lin, A.I., Torino, G.C. & Rivera, D.P. (2007b). Racial microaggressions against black Americans: Implications for counseling. *Journal of Counseling and Development*, Summer 86(3): 330–338. doi: https://doi.org/10.1002/j.1556-6678.2008.tb00517.x

Sullivan, A.L. & A'Vant, E. (2009). Multicultural affairs: On the need for cultural responsiveness. *Communique*, 38(3): 8–9. ISSN: ISSN-0164-775X

Suyemoto, K.L., Hochman, A.L., Donovan, R.A. & Roemer, L. (2020). Becoming and fostering allied and accomplices through authentic relationships: Choosing justice over comfort. *Research in Human Development*, 1–27. doi: https://doi.org/10.1080/15427609.2020.1825905

Talero, P., Kern, S.B. & Tupé, D.A. (2015). Culturally responsive care in occupational therapy: An entry-level educational model embedded in service-learning. *Scandinavian Journal of Occupational Therapy*, 22(2): 95–102. doi: https://doi.org/10.3109/11038128.2014.997287

Tate, W.F. (1997). Critical Race Theory and Education: History, Theory and Implications. In M.W. Apple (ed.), *Review of Research in Education* (pp.195–247). Washington, DC: American Educational Research Association

Tawney, R.H. (1983). *Equality.* London: George Unwin Allen Ltd. (Original work published 1931)

Tehrani, N. (2015). Why is my curriculum white? *Occupied Times*, 27 August. Available at: https://theoccupiedtimes.org/?p=14056 accessed 10 February 2023

The Guardian. (2021). *Police killings of Black Americans amount to crimes against humanity, international inquiry finds.* Available at: www.theguardian.com/us-news/2021/apr/26/us-police-killings-black-americans-crimes-against-humanity accessed 11 February 2023

The Health Foundation. (2021). *Inequalities.* Available at: www.health.org.uk/topics/inequalities accessed 20 December 2021

Thomas, A. (2017). *The Hate U Give* (first edition). New York, NY: Balzer + Bray

Thomas, C. (2022). *The Five Health Frontiers, A New Radial Blueprint.* London: Pluto Press

Thomas, D. (2020). Don't let the pandemic overshadow racial inequalities in higher education. *Times Higher Education Supplement.* Available at: www.timeshighereducation.com/blog/dont-let-the-pandemic-overshadow-racial-inequalities-higher-education accessed 12 December 2021

Thomas, L., Hill, M., Mahony, J.O. & Yorke, M. (2017). *What Works Student Retention and Success Programme. Supporting student success: strategies for institutional change: final report.* Available at: www.advance-he.ac.uk/knowledge-hub/supporting-student-success-strategies-institutional-change accessed 31 May 2021

Thong, T. (2012). To raise the savage to a higher level: The westernization of Nagas and their culture. *Modern Asian Studies*, 46(4): 893–891. doi: https://doi.org/10.1017/S0026749X11000412

Tolliver, M. (2020). *Becoming Anti-Racist.* John T. Milliken Department of Medicine. Available at: https://internalmedicine.wustl.edu/becoming-anti-racist accessed 15 June 2021

Torres, L., Driscoll, M.W. & Burrow, A.L. (2010). Racial microaggressions and psychological functioning among highly achieving African-Americans: A mixed-methods approach. *Journal of Social and Clinical Psychology*, 29(10): 1074–1099. doi: https://doi.org/10.1521/jscp.2010.29.10.1074

Townsend, E. & Polatajko, H.J., Canadian Association of Occupational Therapists. (2007). *Enabling occupation II: Advancing an occupational therapy vision for health, well-being & justice through occupation.* Ottawa, Canada: Canadian Association of Occupational Therapists Publications

Townsend, E. & Whiteford, G. (2005). A Participatory Occupational Justice Framework: Population Based Processes of Practice. In F. Kronenberg, S.S. Algado & N. Pollard (eds), *Occupational Therapy Without Borders* (pp.110–126). Edinburgh: Churchill Livingstone Elsevier

Townsend, E. & Wilcock, A. (2004a). Occupational justice and client-centred practice: A dialogue in progress. *Canadian Journal of Occupational Therapy*, 71(2): 75–87. doi: https://doi.org/10.1177/000841740407100203

Townsend, E.A. & Wilcock, A. (2004b). Occupational Justice. In C. Christiansen & E. Townsend, *Introduction to Occupation: The Art and Science of Living* (pp.243–273). Upper Saddle River, NJ: Prentice-Hall

Trentham, B., Cockburn, L., Cameron, D. & Iwama, M. (2007). Diversity and inclusion within an occupational therapy curriculum. *Australian Occupational Therapy Journal*, 54(s1): S49–S57. doi: https://doi.org/10.1111/j.1440-1630.2006.00605.x

Turcotte, P.-L. & Holmes, D. (2021). The (dis)obedient occupational therapist: A reflection on dissent against disciplinary propaganda. *Cadernos Brasileiros de Terapia Ocupacional*, 29, e2924. doi: https://doi.org/10.1590/2526-8910.ctoARF2211

Turner, A. & Knight, J. (2015). A debate on the professional identity of occupational therapists. *British Journal of Occupational Therapy*, 78(11): 664–673. doi: https://doi.org/10.1177/0308022615601439

Tutu, D. & Van Roekel, D. (2010). Facing the Future: Global Education at the Crossroads. *Huffington Post*. Available at: www.huffpost.com/entry/facing-the-future-global_b_544449 accessed 15 June 2022

Tyldesley, B. (2004). Alice Constance Owens – reflections upon a remarkable lady and a pioneer of occupational therapy in England. *British Journal of Occupational Therapy*, 67(11): 165–173. doi: https://doi.org/10.1177/030802260406711S123

UNESCO. (2003). *Text of the Convention for the Safeguarding of the Intangible Cultural Heritage*, Paris, 29 September to 17 October. Available at: https://ich.unesco.org/en/convention accessed 8 January 2020

Universities UK and National Union of Students. (2019). *Black, Asian and minority ethnic student attainment at UK university #Closingthegap.* Available at: www.universitiesuk.ac.uk/policy-and-analysis/reports/Documents/2019/bame-student-attainment-uk-universities-closing-the-gap.pdf accessed 15 October 2020

University College London. (2020). *BAME Award Gap Project – Staff Toolkit.* Available at: www.ucl.ac.uk/teaching-learning/sites/teaching-learning/files/bame_awarding_gap_toolkit_2020.pdf accessed 31 May 2021

Uys, K. & Samuels, A. (2010). Early Childhood Intervention in South Africa: Minimising the Impact of Disabilities. In V. Alers & R. Crouch (eds), *Occupational Therapy: An African Perspective* (pp.206–231). Johannesberg, SA: Sarah Shorten

Vachon, W. & McConnell, T. (2018). Allies, Not Accomplices: What Youth Work Can Learn from Trans and Disability Movements. In *The SAGE Handbook of Youth Work Practice* (pp.426–438). London: Sage Publications

van Vuuren, J.J., Okyere, C. & Aldersey, H. (2020). The role of occupational therapy in Africa: A scoping review. *South African Journal of Occupational Therapy*, 50(3): 3–21. doi: https://doi.org/10.1080/09638288.2020.1743779

Walder, K., Bissett, M., Molineux, M. & Whiteford, G. (2022). Understanding professional identity in occupational therapy: A scoping review. *Scandinavian Journal of Occupational Therapy*, 29(3), 175–197. doi: https://doi.org/10.1080/11038128.2021.1974548

Wane, N.N. & Todd, K.L. (2018). *Decolonial Pedagogy: Examining Sites of Resistance, Resurgence, and Renewal.* Switzerland: Pelgrave Macmillan, Springer International Publishing

Warmington, P. (2019). Critical race theory in England: Impact and opposition. *Global Studies in Culture and Power*, 27(1): 20–37. doi: https://doi.org/10.1080/1070289X.2019.1587907

Watson, R. (2006). Being before doing: The cultural identity (essence) of occupational therapy. *Australian Journal of Occupational Therapy*, 53: 151–158. doi: https://doi.org/10.1111/j.1440-1630.2006.00598.x

West, C. (1995). Foreword. In K. Crenshaw, N. Gotanda, G. Peller & K. Thomas (eds), *Critical Race Theory: The Key Writings that Formed the Movement* (pp.xi–xii). New York, NY: New Press

Whalley Hammell, K.R. (2017). Opportunities for well-being: The right to occupational engagement. *Canadian Journal of Occupational Therapy*, 84(4–5): 209–222. doi: https://doi.org/10.1177/0008417417734831

Whalley Hammell, K.R. (2019). Building globally relevant occupational therapy from the strength of our diversity. *World Federation of Occupational Therapists Bulletin*, 75(1): 13–26. doi: https://doi.org/10.1080/14473828.2018.1529480

Whalley Hammell, K.R. & Iwama, M.K. (2012). Well-being and occupational rights: An imperative for critical occupational therapy. *Scandinavian Journal of Occupational Therapy*, 19(5): 385–394. doi: https://doi.org/10.3109/11038128.2011.611821

Whiteford, G. & Townsend, E. (2010). Participatory Occupational Justice Framework (POJF) 2010: Enabling Occupational Participation and Inclusion. In F. Kronenberg, N. Pollard & D. Sakellariou (eds), *Occupational Therapies Without Borders* (pp.65–84). Edinburgh: Churchill Livingstone Elsevier

References

Whiteford, G. & Wilcock, A. (2000). Cultural Relativism: occupational and independence reconsidered. *Canadian Journal of Occupational Therapy*, 67: 324–336. doi: https://doi.org/10.1177/000841740006700505

Wilcock, A.A. (2006). *An Occupational Perspective of Health* (second edition). Thorofare, NJ: Slack

Wilcock, A.A. & Hocking, C. (2015). *An Occupational Perspective of Health* (third edition). Thorofare, NJ: Slack

Wilcock, A. & Townsend, E. (2000). Occupational terminology interactive dialogue. *Journal of Occupational Science*, 7(2): 84–86. doi: https://doi.org/10.1080/14427591.2000.9686470

Wilcock, A.A. & Townsend, E.A. (2009). Occupational Justice. In E.B. Crepeau, E.S. Cohn & B.A. Boyt Schell (eds), *Willard & Spackman's Occupational Therapy* (11th edition) (pp.192–199). Baltimore, MD: Lippincott Williams & Wilkins

Wilkerson, I. (2020). *Caste: The Lies that Divide Us*. New York, NY: Random House

Willer-Kherbaoui, J. (2019). Working through the smog: How white individuals develop critical consciousness of white saviorism. *Community Engagement Student Work*, 29. Available at: https://scholarworks.merrimack.edu/soe_student_ce/29 23 accessed June 2022

Williams, D. (2016). *How racism makes us sick*. Available at: www.youtube.com/watch?v=Vzy-jDR_AWzE accessed 9 March 2022

Williams, D. (2019). *King's Fund Podcast: On Racism, Discrimination and the Impact They Have on Health*. Available at: http://kingsfund.libsyn.com/professor-david-williams-on-racism-discrimination-and-the-impact-it-has-on-health accessed 31 December 2021

Williams, D.R., Lawrence, J.A. & Davis, B.A. (2019). Racism and health: Evidence and needed research. *Annual Review of Public Health*, 1(40): 105–125. doi: https://doi.org/10.1146/annurev-publhealth-040218-043750

Williams, D. & Rucker, T. (2000). Understanding and addressing racial disparities in health care. *Health Care Financing Review*, 21(4): 75–90

Williams, D.R. & Mohammed, S.A. (2013). Racism and Health 1: Pathways and scientific evidence. *American Behavioral Scientist*, 57(8). doi: https://doi.org/10.1177/0002764213487340

Williams, D.R. & Purdie-Vaughns, V. (2016). Needed interventions to reduce racial/ethnic disparities in health. *Journal of Health Politics Policy and Law*, 41: 627–651. doi: https://doi.org/10.1215/03616878-3620857

Williams, E., Buck, D. & Babalola, G. (2020). *What are health inequalities*. Available at: www.kingsfund.org.uk/publications/what-are-health-inequalities accessed 20 December 2021

Williams, E. & De Witt, P.A. (2020). Guest editorial. *South African Journal of Occupational Therapy*, 50(2): 2–3. Available at: https://sajot.org.za/index.php/sajot/issue/view/39 accessed 11 February 2023

Williams, J. & Romer, C. (2020). *In U.S. Counties where Lynchings were prevalent, police are more likely to shoot Black people*. Available at: https://inthesetimes.com/article/police-killings-black-lives-matter-lynchings-george-floyd accessed 31 December 2021

Wingfield, A.H. & Alston, R.S. (2014). Maintaining hierarchies in predominantly white organizations. *American Behavioral Scientist*, 58(2): 274–287, doi: https://doi.org/10.1177/0002764213503329

Woodall, J., South, J., Dixey, R., De Viggiani, N. & Penson, W. (2015). Factors that determine the effectiveness of peer interventions in prisons in England and Wales. *Prison Service Journal*, May issue 219: 30–37. Available at: www.crimeandjustice.org.uk/publications/psj/prison-service-journal-219 accessed 9 July 2022

World Federation of Occupational Therapists (WFOT). (2010). *Definition 'Occupation'*. Available at: https://wfot.org/about/about-occupational-therapy#:~:text=Definition%20%20Occupation%22,and%20are%20expected%20to%20do accessed 14 April 2021

World Federation of Occupational Therapists (WFOT). (2016). *Minimum Standards for the Education of Occupational Therapists*. Available at: www.wfot.org/assets/resources/COPYRIGHTED-World-Federation-of-Occupational-Therapists-Minimum-Standards-for-the-Education-of-Occupational-Therapists-2016a.pdf accessed 30 July 2021

World Federation of Occupational Therapists (WFOT). (2019). *Occupational Therapy and Human Rights.* Available at: https://wfot.org/resources/occupational-therapy-and-human-rights accessed 22 December 2021

World Federation of Occupational Therapists (WFOT). (2020). *Statement on Systemic Racism.* Available at: www.wfot.org/resources/wfot-statement-on-systemic-racism accessed 27 March 2021

World Federation of Occupational Therapists (WFOT). (2021). *About Occupational Therapy.* Available at: https://wfot.org/about/about-occupational-therapy accessed 22 December 2021

World Health Organization (WHO). (1999). *Health 21: The Health For All Policy Framework for the WHO European Region.* Copenhagen, Denmark: World Health Organization

World Health Organization (WHO). (2018). *Health Inequities and their Causes.* Available at: www.who.int/news-room/facts-in-pictures/detail/health-inequities-and-their-causes accessed 12 October 2021

World Health Organization (WHO). (2021). *World Health Organization Social Determinants of Health.* Available at: www.who.int/health-topics/social-determinants-of-health#tab=tab_1 accessed 12 October 2021

World Health Organization (WHO). (2022). *Constitution of World Health Organization 1946.* World Health Organization. Available at: www.who.int/about/governance/constitution accessed 8 October 2022

Yañez, R. & Zúñiga, Y. (2018). The law and occupational justice: Inputs for the understanding of disability in Chile. *Journal of Occupational Science*, 25(4): 520–529. doi: https://doi.org/10.1080/14427591.2018.1522945

Yeager, K.A. & Bauer-Wu, S. (2013). Cultural humility: Essential foundation for clinical researchers. *Applied Nursing Research*, Nov, 26(4): 1–12. doi: https://doi.org/10.1016/j.apnr.2013.06.008

Yu, C. (2021). An examination of the institutionally oppressive white savior complex in Uganda through western documentaries. *International Social Science Review*, 97(2). Available at: https://go.gale.com/ps/i.do?id=GALE%7CA668019184&sid=googleScholar&v=2.1&it=r&linkaccess=abs&issn=02782308&p=AONE&sw=w&userGroupName=anon%7Ece1e419d accessed 10 February 2023

Subject Index

Author Index